50 Studies Every Vascular Surgeon Should Know

50 STUDIES EVERY DOCTOR SHOULD KNOW

50 Studies Every Doctor Should Know: The Key Studies that Form the Foundation of Evidence Based Medicine, Revised Edition
Michael E. Hochman

50 Studies Every Internist Should Know
Kristopher Swiger, Joshua R. Thomas, Michael E. Hochman, and Steven Hochman

50 Studies Every Neurologist Should Know
David Y. Hwang and David M. Greer

50 Studies Every Pediatrician Should Know
Ashaunta T. Anderson, Nina L. Shapiro, Stephen C. Aronoff, Jeremiah Davis, and Michael Levy

50 Imaging Studies Every Doctor Should Know
Christoph I. Lee

50 Studies Every Surgeon Should Know
SreyRam Kuy, Rachel J. Kwon, and Miguel A. Burch

50 Studies Every Intensivist Should Know
Edward A. Bittner

50 Studies Every Palliative Care Doctor Should Know
David Hui, Akhila Reddy, and Eduardo Bruera

50 Studies Every Psychiatrist Should Know
Ish P. Bhalla, Rajesh R. Tampi, and Vinod H. Srihari

50 Studies Every Anesthesiologist Should Know
Anita Gupta, Michael E. Hochman, and Elena N. Gutman

50 Studies Every Ophthalmologist Should Know
Alan D. Penman, Kimberly W. Crowder, and William M. Watkins, Jr.

50 Studies Every Urologist Should Know
Philipp Dahm

50 Studies Every Obstetrician and Gynecologist Should Know
Constance Liu, Noah Rindos, and Scott Shainker

50 Studies Every Doctor Should Know: The Key Studies that Form the Foundation of Evidence-Based Medicine, 2nd Edition
Michael E. Hochman and Steven D. Hochman

50 Studies Every Occupational Therapist Should Know
Elizabeth A. Pyatak and Elissa S. Lee

50 Studies Every Vascular Surgeon Should Know
Julien Al Shakarchi

50 Studies Every Vascular Surgeon Should Know

EDITED BY

JULIEN AL SHAKARCHI
Consultant Vascular Surgeon
Department of Vascular Surgery
Worcestershire Acute Hospitals NHS Trust
Worcester, UK

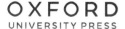

OXFORD
UNIVERSITY PRESS

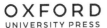

Oxford University Press is a department of the University of Oxford. It furthers the University's objective of excellence in research, scholarship, and education by publishing worldwide. Oxford is a registered trade mark of Oxford University Press in the UK and certain other countries.

Published in the United States of America by Oxford University Press
198 Madison Avenue, New York, NY 10016, United States of America.

CIP data is on file at the Library of Congress

ISBN 978-0-19-763790-6

DOI: 10.1093/med/9780197637906.001.0001

9 8 7 6 5 4 3 2 1

Printed by Marquis, Canada

To Neba, Adam and Faith for your endless support and love.

– Julien Al Shakarchi

CONTENTS

SECTION 3 Thoracic Outlet

Julien Al Shakarchi and Andrew Garnham

SECTION 4 Thoracic Aortic Disease

Julien Al Shakarchi and Donald Adam

SECTION 8 Venous Disease

Julien Al Shakarchi and Isaac Nyamekye

SECTION 9 Vascular Access

Julien Al Shakarchi and Nicholas Inston

SECTION 10 Trauma

Julien Al Shakarchi and Jack Fairhead

CONTRIBUTORS

Donald Adam, MBChB, FRCS, MD
University Hospitals Birmingham
Birmingham, UK

**Julien Al Shakarchi, MBChB, FRCS
(vasc), MD**
Worcestershire Acute Hospitals
  NHS Trust
Worcester, UK

Richard Downing, BSc, MD, FRCS
Worcestershire Royal Hospital
Worcester, UK

Jack Fairhead, MBChB, FRCS
University Hospitals of North Midlands
Stoke-on-Trent, UK

Andrew Garnham, MB, BCH, FRCS
Wolverhampton NHS Trust, Black
  Country Vascular Unit
Wolverhampton, UK

**Nicholas Inston, MBChB,
FRCS, PhD**
University Hospitals Birmingham
Birmingham, UK

**Lewis Meecham, MBChB, FRCS
(vasc), MD**
University Hospital of Wales
Cardiff, UK

**Isaac Nyamekye, MBChB,
FRCS(Eng), MD**
Worcestershire Acute Hospitals
  NHS Trust
Worcester, UK

Alok Tiwari, MBBS, MS, FRCSEd
University Hospitals Birmingham
Birmingham, UK

Secondary Prevention
in Peripheral Arterial Disease

JULIEN AL SHAKARCHI AND ANDREW GARNHAM

1

Clopidogrel Versus Aspirin in Patients at Risk of Ischemic Events (CAPRIE)

A Randomized, Blinded Trial

> Clopidogrel is an effective new antiplatelet agent for use in atherothrombotic disease.
>
> THE CAPRIE INVESTIGATORS

Research Question: Does clopidogrel provide a benefit compared to aspirin in reducing the risk of ischemic stroke, myocardial infarction (MI), or vascular death in patients with recent ischemic stroke, recent MI, or peripheral arterial disease (PAD)?[1]

Funding: Industrial funding from Sanofi and Bristol-Myers Squibb

Year Study Began: 1992

Year Study Published: 1996

Study Location: 384 clinical centers from 16 countries

Who Was Studied: Patients over the age of 21 who had either:
- Recent proven ischemic stroke (onset >1 week, <6 months) likely of atherothrombotic origin
- Recent MI (<35 days)

- Atherosclerotic PAD (intermittent claudication with ankle–brachial pressure index (ABPI) <0.85 or history of intermittent claudication with previous revascularization or amputation)

Who Was Excluded: Patients with uncontrolled hypertension, carotid endarterectomy after qualifying stroke, limited life expectancy (<3 years), scheduled surgery, or contraindication to study drugs (hemostatic disorder or history of, renal/hepatic insufficiency, or hematologic disorder)

Patients: 19,185

Study Overview

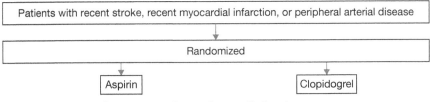

Figure 1.1 Design of CAPRIE randomized controlled trial

Study Intervention: Patients were randomly assigned to a 75-mg clopidogrel tablet with aspirin placebo or a 325-mg aspirin tablet with clopidogrel placebo. Patients were asked to take their tablets daily with their morning meal.

Follow-up: Mean duration of 1.91 years

Endpoints: Primary outcome: Composite of ischemic stroke, MI, or vascular death. *Secondary outcomes:* Composite of ischemic stroke, MI, leg amputation, or vascular death; composite of any stroke, MI, or death from any cause; vascular death; death from any cause.

RESULTS

- 42 patients (0.22%) were lost to follow-up, 22 in the clopidogrel group and 20 in the aspirin group.
- The composite primary outcome (ischemic stroke, MI, or vascular death) was found to be significantly higher in the aspirin group than in the clopidogrel group (Table 1.1).

- There was no significant difference in vascular death, death from any cause, or the composite secondary outcome of ischemic stroke, MI, amputation, or vascular death.
- In the subgroup analysis, the PAD group benefited significantly from the use of clopidogrel but the stroke and MI groups did not (see Table 1.1).
- In terms of severe adverse events, aspirin led to significantly more gastrointestinal hemorrhage and clopidogrel caused more rashes.

Table 1.1 TREATMENT EFFECT BY SUBGROUP—ISCHEMIC STROKE, MI, OR VASCULAR DEATH

Subgroup population	Treatment group	Number of events	Event rate per year	Relative risk reduction (95% CI)	p value
Stroke	Clopidogrel	433	7.15%	7.3% (−5.7 to 18.7)	0.26
	Aspirin	461	7.71%		
MI	Clopidogrel	291	5.03%	−3.7% (−22.1 to 12.0)	0.66
	Aspirin	283	4.84%		
PAD	Clopidogrel	215	3.71%	23.8% (8.9–36.2)	0.0028
	Aspirin	277	4.86%		
Overall	Clopidogrel	939	5.32%	8.7% (0.3–16.5)	0.043
	Aspirin	1,021	5.83%		

CI, confidence interval.

Criticisms and Limitations: The use of composite outcomes has been criticized as it is easy for readers to assume mistakenly that the treatment effect applies to all components. However, the number of patients required to power the study for each outcome individually would have been challenging and costly. Also, there is little information on concomitant medications, such as statins, that may have confounded the outcomes.

Other Relevant Studies and Information

- The Clopidogrel for High Atherothrombotic Risk and Ischemic Stabilization, Management, and Avoidance (CHARISMA) trial assigned patients with either clinically evident cardiovascular disease or multiple risk factors to receive dual therapy or aspirin alone. In the overall population dual therapy provided no additional benefit.[2] However, in patients with prior MI, stroke, or symptomatic PAD, there was a reduced rate of the composite outcome of stroke, MI, or death.[3]

- The Clopidogrel and Acetylsalicylic Acid in Bypass Surgery for Peripheral Arterial Disease (CASPAR) trial looked at the use of dual therapy following below-knee bypass surgery and found no evidence of improved outcomes (composite of graft occlusion/revascularization, major amputation, or death). However, in a subgroup analysis, there was benefit in patients receiving prosthetic grafts.[4]
- The Clopidogrel with Aspirin in Acute Minor Stroke or Transient Ischemic Attack (CHANCE) trial showed a reduction in stroke rate with dual antiplatelet therapy in the first 90 days following a stroke or transient ischemic attack.[5]
- The Global Vascular Guidelines on the management of chronic limb-threatening ischemia (CLTI) recommend clopidogrel as the single antiplatelet agent of choice in patients with CLTI.[6]

Summary and Implications: For patients with vascular disease, the CAPRIE trial found clopidogrel to be a safe and efficacious antiplatelet agent, marginally better than aspirin for preventing subsequent vascular events. Clopidogrel is now a well-established treatment for vascular disease and is recommended as the antiplatelet agent of choice in patients with PAD.

CLINICAL CASE: ANTIPLATELET THERAPY FOR PAD

Case History
A family doctor asks your expert opinion for a 75-year-old man with a history of intermittent claudication. The patient has a claudication distance of 250 meters and his quality of life is unaffected by this. He is an ex-smoker and currently takes aspirin. He would like advice on the antiplatelet of choice for his patient.

Suggested Answer
Among patients with PAD, the CAPRIE trial showed a relative risk reduction of 23.8% in the composite outcome of ischemic stroke, MI, or vascular death. In view of this and the history given, the family doctor should be advised to change aspirin to clopidogrel unless there is a contraindication. The patient does not require any intervention for his claudication as his quality of life is unaffected; however, he should be offered a supervised exercise program to improve his walking distance.

References

1. Gent M, Beaumont D, Blanchard J, et al. A randomised, blinded trial of Clopidogrel versus Aspirin in Patients at Risk of Ischaemic Events (CAPRIE). *Lancet.* 1996;348(9038):1329–1339.
2. CHARISMA Investigators. Clopidogrel and aspirin versus aspirin alone for the prevention of atherothrombotic events. *N Engl J Med.* 2006;354(16):1706–1717.
3. CHARISMA Investigators. Patients with prior myocardial infarction, stroke, or symptomatic peripheral arterial disease in the CHARISMA trial. *J Am Coll Cardiol.* 2007;49(19):1982–1988.
4. CASPAR Writing Committee. Results of the randomized, placebo-controlled Clopidogrel and Acetylsalicylic Acid in Bypass Surgery for Peripheral Arterial Disease (CASPAR) trial. *J Vasc Surg.* 2010;52(4):825–833.
5. CHANCE Investigators. Clopidogrel with Aspirin in Acute Minor Stroke or Transient Ischemic Attack (CHANCE) trial: One-year outcomes. *Circulation.* 2015;132(1):40–46.
6. GVG Writing Group for the Joint Guidelines of the Society for Vascular Surgery (SVS), European Society for Vascular Surgery (ESVS), and World Federation of Vascular Societies (WFVS). Global vascular guidelines on the management of chronic limb-threatening ischemia. *Eur J Vasc Endovasc Surg.* 2019;58(1S):S1–S109.

2

Rivaroxaban With or Without Aspirin in Patients with Stable Peripheral or Carotid Artery Disease

Cardiovascular Outcomes for People Using Anticoagulation Strategies (COMPASS), an International, Randomized, Double-Blind, Placebo-Controlled Trial

The combination of rivaroxaban and aspirin represents an important advance in the management of patients with peripheral artery disease.

THE COMPASS INVESTIGATORS

Research Question: Does rivaroxaban with or without aspirin provide a benefit compared to aspirin in reducing the risk of ischemic stroke, myocardial infarction (MI), or vascular death in patients with stable peripheral or carotid arterial disease?[1]

Funding: Industrial funding from Bayer

Year Study Began: 2013

Year Study Published: 2018

Study Location: 602 clinical centers from 33 countries

Who Was Studied: Patients had either:

- Peripheral artery disease defined by any one of the following: aortofemoral bypass surgery, limb bypass surgery, percutaneous transluminal angioplasty revascularization of the iliac or infrainguinal arteries; or limb or foot amputation for arterial vascular disease; or intermittent claudication and one or more of either an ankle–brachial index (ABI) of <0.90 or a peripheral artery stenosis (≥50%) documented by angiography or duplex ultrasound
- Carotid revascularization or asymptomatic carotid artery stenosis of ≥50% diagnosed by duplex ultrasound or angiography.
- Coronary artery disease with an ABI of <0.90 were included in the overall peripheral artery disease cohort.

Who Was Excluded: Patients with a high risk of bleeding, stroke within 1 month, a history of hemorrhagic or lacunar stroke, severe heart failure with a known ejection fraction of <30%, or estimated glomerular filtration rate of <15 ml/min

Patients: 7,470

Study Overview

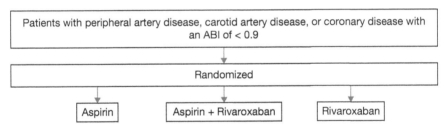

Figure 2.1 Design of COMPASS randomized controlled trial

Study Intervention: After a 30-day run-in period, eligible patients were randomly assigned to receive 100 mg aspirin once a day, aspirin 100 mg one a day with low-dose rivaroxaban 2.5 mg twice a day, or rivaroxaban 5 mg twice a day.

Follow-up: Mean duration of 21 months

Endpoints: The primary outcome was cardiovascular death, MI, or stroke. The peripheral artery disease outcome was major adverse limb events, including major amputation.

RESULTS

- 6,048 participants with peripheral or carotid artery disease were enrolled and an additional 1,422 patients were enrolled with coronary artery disease who had an ABI <0.9.
- 5 patients (0.06%) were lost to follow-up.
- The composite primary outcome (ischemic stroke, MI, or vascular death) was found to be significantly different between the groups: 5% in the low-dose rivaroxaban + aspirin group compared to 6% in the rivaroxaban group and 7% in the aspirin group (Table 2.1).
- The rate of major adverse limb events including amputation was found to be significantly different between the groups: 1% in the low-dose rivaroxaban + aspirin group compared to 2% in the rivaroxaban group and 2% in the aspirin group.
- The rate of major adverse cardiovascular and limb events including amputation was found to be significantly different between the groups: 6% in the low-dose rivaroxaban + aspirin group compared to 8% in the rivaroxaban group and 9% in the aspirin group.
- Major bleeding occurred in 3% of patients who took low-dose rivaroxaban + aspirin, 3% of patients who took rivaroxaban alone, and 2% of patients who took aspirin alone. No differences in fatal bleeding or nonfatal intracranial hemorrhages were observed between the three different groups.

Table 2.1 EVENT RATE OF OUTCOME MEASURES PER TREATMENT GROUPS

Outcome measure	Low-dose rivaroxaban + aspirin (n = 2,492)	Rivaroxaban alone (n = 2,474)	Aspirin alone (n = 2,504)
Cardiovascular death, stroke, or MI	126 (5%)	149 (6%)	174 (7%)
MI	51 (2%)	56 (2%)	67 (3%)
Stroke	25 (1%)	43 (2%)	47 (2%)
Cardiovascular death	64 (3%)	66 (3%)	78 (3%)
Major adverse limb event	30 (1%)	35 (1%)	56 (2%)

Criticisms and Limitations: The main criticism of the trial was that aspirin was used as a comparator rather than clopidogrel. The Clopidogrel Versus Aspirin in Patients at Risk of Ischaemic events (CAPRIE) trial (see Chapter 1) has shown that clopidogrel reduce major adverse cardiac events when compared to aspirin.[2] In addition, unlike the CAPRIE trial, which found clopidogrel not to have any added adverse events, the addition of low-dose rivaroxaban does increase the risk of bleeding.

In addition, exclusion of participants after the run-in period due to adherence issues raises the possibility of selection bias, and therefore results might be different in clinical practice. ABI was measured using a sphygmomanometer and palpation of the artery in most individuals, which is unusual in vascular practice.

Other Relevant Studies and Information

- Rivaroxaban is a new-generation anticoagulant and acts by inhibiting factor Xa in the coagulation cascade. Over the last decade, use of factor Xa inhibitors has increased dramatically, and they have replaced vitamin K antagonists as the first-choice anticoagulant in various clinical scenarios.
- The EINSTEIN study compared rivaroxaban with subcutaneous enoxaparin followed by warfarin in the treatment of acute deep vein thrombosis. It found this new drug to be non-inferior and safe.[3]
- The Rivaroxaban Once Daily Oral Direct Factor Xa Inhibition Compared with Vitamin K Antagonism for Prevention of Stroke and Embolism Trial in Atrial Fibrillation (ROCKET AF) study, a randomized controlled trial, compared rivaroxaban to warfarin in patients with atrial fibrillation. Rivaroxaban was found to be non-inferior to warfarin for the prevention of stroke and systemic embolization.[4]
- In contrast to the benefits seen in this study with combination rivaroxaban and aspirin, studies have suggested that combination vitamin K antagonists with antiplatelet do not provide any benefit in terms of major adverse cardiac events when compared to antiplatelet alone, but they do increase bleeding risk.[5]
- The Global Vascular Guidelines on the management of chronic limb-threatening ischemia (CLTI) recommend considering low-dose aspirin and rivaroxaban, 2.5 mg twice a day, to reduce adverse cardiovascular events and lower extremity ischemic events in patients with CLTI.[6]

Summary and Implications: In patients with established carotid and peripheral artery disease, rivaroxaban plus aspirin resulted in a 2% absolute risk reduction in cardiovascular death, stroke, or nonfatal MI and a 1% absolute risk reduction in major limb event including amputation. This benefit was partially offset by a 1% increased absolute risk in major bleeding.

CLINICAL CASE: ANTIPLATELET THERAPY FOR PERIPHERAL ARTERIAL DISEASE

Case History

A 70-year-old man with a previous history of an iliac angioplasty attends your outpatient clinic. He would like advice on the best management of his cardio-vascular risk. He is currently taking aspirin and atorvastatin.

Suggested Answer

The COMPASS trial has shown that if the patient has a low risk of bleeding and does not have any other contraindication he should be offered low-dose rivaroxaban in addition to his aspirin. The combination of these two drugs provides a reduction of both major cardiovascular and limb events.

References

1. COMPASS Investigators. Rivaroxaban with or without aspirin in patients with stable peripheral or carotid artery disease: An international, randomised, double-blind, placebo-controlled trial. *Lancet.* 2018;391(10117):219–229.
2. Gent M, Beaumont D, Blanchard J, et al. A randomised, blinded trial of Clopidogrel Versus Aspirin in Patients at Risk of Ischaemic Events (CAPRIE). *Lancet.* 1996;348(9038):1329–1339.
3. EINSTEIN Investigators. Oral rivaroxaban for symptomatic venous thromboembolism. *N Engl J Med.* 2010;363(26):2499–2510.
4. ROCKET AF Investigators. Rivaroxaban versus warfarin in nonvalvular atrial fibrillation. *N Engl J Med.* 2011;365(10):883–891.
5. WAVE Investigators. Oral anticoagulant and antiplatelet therapy and peripheral arterial disease. *N Engl J Med.* 2007;357(3):217–227.
6. GVG Writing Group for the Joint Guidelines of the Society for Vascular Surgery (SVS), European Society for Vascular Surgery (ESVS), and World Federation of Vascular Societies (WFVS). Global vascular guidelines on the management of chronic limb-threatening ischemia. *Eur J Vasc Endovasc Surg.* 2019;58(1S):S1–S109.

3

Rivaroxaban in Peripheral Artery Disease After Revascularization (VOYAGER)

The benefit was apparent early, with the Kaplan–Meier curves separating at 3 months.

THE VOYAGER INVESTIGATORS

Research Question: Does rivaroxaban with aspirin provide a benefit compared to aspirin alone in reducing the risk of acute limb ischemia, amputation, ischemic stroke, myocardial infarction (MI), or vascular death in patients who have undergone revascularization?[1]

Funding: Industrial funding from Bayer and Janssen

Year Study Began: 2015

Year Study Published: 2020

Study Location: 542 clinical centers from 34 countries

Who Was Studied: Patients, at least 50 years of age, were eligible after a successful revascularization within the last 10 days for symptoms of peripheral arterial disease (PAD). Patients were required to have documented lower-extremity PAD, including symptoms, anatomic evidence, and hemodynamic evidence.

Who Was Excluded: Patients were excluded from the study if their clinical condition was unstable, if they were at a heightened risk for bleeding, or if they were taking or were anticipated to begin taking prohibited concomitant medications, including long-term treatment with clopidogrel.

Patients: 6,564

Study Overview

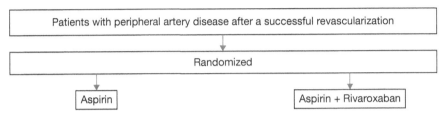

Figure 3.1 Design of VOYAGER randomized controlled trial

Study Intervention: In this randomized controlled trial, eligible patients were randomly assigned to receive 100 mg aspirin once a day with placebo twice a day or aspirin 100 mg once a day with low-dose rivaroxaban 2.5 mg twice a day.

Follow-up: Mean duration of 28 months

Endpoints: The primary outcome was a composite of acute limb ischemia, amputation, MI, stroke, or cardiovascular death. The principal safety outcome was major bleeding defined according to the Thrombolysis in Myocardial Infarction (TIMI) classification.

RESULTS

- The majority of patients had a history of claudication (77%), while the rest had critical limb ischemia (23%). Approximately two thirds of patients had been treated with an endovascular procedure (65%), and one third had been treated surgically (35%).
- Only 6 patients (0.09%) were lost to follow-up. However, 1,080 patients (33.2%) in the rivaroxaban group and 1,011 patients (31.1%) in the placebo group discontinued treatment prematurely.
- The composite primary outcome (acute limb ischemia, amputation, ischemic stroke, MI, or vascular death) was found to be significantly different between the groups. It occurred in the low-dose rivaroxaban +

aspirin group in 15.5% of patients, compared to 17.8% in the aspirin-alone
group (Table 3.1).
• The rate of unplanned revascularization for recurrent event was also
  significantly different, at 17.8% in the low-dose rivaroxaban + aspirin
  group compared to 20% in the aspirin-alone group.
• The rate of TIMI major bleeding was not found to be significantly different
  between the two groups (1.9% in the rivaroxaban + aspirin group, 1.35%
  in the aspirin-only group).

Table 3.1 EVENT RATE OF OUTCOME MEASURES PER TREATMENT GROUPS

Outcome measure	Low-dose rivaroxaban + aspirin (n = 3,286)	Placebo + aspirin (n = 3,278)	p value
Acute limb ischemia, amputation, MI, stroke, or cardiovascular death	508 (15.5%)	584 (17.8%)	0.009
Acute limb ischemia	155 (4.7%)	227 (6.9%)	
Amputation	103 (3.1%)	115 (3.5%)	
MI	131 (4.0%)	148 (4.5%)	
Stroke	71 (2.2%)	82 (2.5%)	
Cardiovascular death	199 (6.1%)	174 (5.3%)	
Unplanned index-limb revascularization for recurrent limb ischemia	584 (17.8%)	655 (20.0%)	0.03

Criticisms and Limitations: The choice of aspirin as comparator treatment in
the VOYAGER PAD trial has been criticized. Clopidogrel, which has been shown
to be a more potent drug than aspirin for secondary prevention, would have been
the more appropriate choice for many clinicians.

An important limitation of the trial is the high percentage of patients who discontinued treatment prematurely, although it was relatively balanced between
the groups. This questions whether the findings can be generalized to clinical
practice.

Rivaroxaban + aspirin was associated with a similar frequency of TIMI major
bleeding; however, there was an increased incidence of International Society on
Thrombosis and Hemostasis (ISTH) major bleeding with rivaroxaban + aspirin
compared with placebo + aspirin.

Other Relevant Studies and Information: Other important studies assessing the use of antiplatelet and anticoagulation therapies for improving outcomes and graft patency following peripheral arterial bypass surgery include:

- A Cochrane review investigated the use of antiplatelet agents for preventing thrombosis after peripheral arterial bypass surgery. It found that aspirin had a beneficial effect on primary patency of peripheral bypass grafts compared to placebo or no treatment.[2]
- The Clopidogrel and Acetylsalicylic Acid in Bypass Surgery for Peripheral Arterial Disease (CASPAR) trial looked at the use of dual therapy following below-knee bypass surgery and found no evidence of improved outcomes (composite of graft occlusion/revascularization, major amputation, or death). However, in a subgroup analysis, there was benefit in patients receiving prosthetic grafts.[3]
- The Dutch Bypass Oral Anticoagulants or Aspirin study randomized 2,690 patients who had undergone infra-inguinal grafting with either anticoagulation or aspirin. In terms of overall graft occlusion, no overall advantage for either treatment was found.[4]

The UK National Institute for Health and Care Excellence (NICE) guidelines recommend rivaroxaban + aspirin as an option for preventing atherothrombotic events in adults with symptomatic PAD who are at high risk of ischemic events.[5]

Summary and Implications: Among patients with lower-extremity PAD undergoing revascularization, rivaroxaban + aspirin was associated with a reduction in major adverse limb and cardiovascular events compared with placebo + aspirin. Benefit for rivaroxaban + aspirin versus placebo + aspirin was similar for endovascular and surgical lower-extremity revascularization, and for revascularization of critical limb ischemia and noncritical limb ischemia. The VOYAGER and Cardiovascular Outcomes for People Using Anticoagulation Strategies (COMPASS; see Chapter 2) trials have shown the benefit of low-dose rivaroxaban with aspirin in PAD patients.[6]

CLINICAL CASE: SECONDARY PREVENTION FOLLOWING INTERVENTION FOR PAD

Case History

A 68-year-old man is admitted to the hospital with critical limb ischemia. He undergoes a femoropopliteal bypass with ipsilateral great saphenous vein. Prior to admission, he was only taking atorvastatin. What medications would you start on this patient?

Suggested Answer

The VOYAGER trial has shown that if the patient has a low risk of bleeding and does not have any other contraindication, he should be offered low-dose rivaroxaban with aspirin. The combination of these two drugs was shown in this trial to lead to a reduction of both major adverse limb and cardiovascular events.

References

1. Bonaca MP, Bauersachs RM, Anand SS, et al. Rivaroxaban in peripheral artery disease after revascularization. *N Engl J Med.* 2020;382(21):1994–2004.
2. Bedenis R, Lethaby A, Maxwell H, et al. Antiplatelet agents for preventing thrombosis after peripheral arterial bypass surgery. *Cochrane Database Syst Rev.* 2015:CD000535.
3. CASPAR Writing Committee. Results of the randomized, placebo-controlled Clopidogrel and Acetylsalicylic Acid in Bypass Surgery for Peripheral Arterial Disease (CASPAR) trial. *J Vasc Surg.* 2010;52(4):825–833.
4. BOA Investigators. Efficacy of oral anticoagulants compared with aspirin after infrainguinal bypass surgery (The Dutch Bypass Oral Anticoagulants or Aspirin Study): A randomised trial. *Lancet.* 2000;355(9201):346–351.
5. National Institute for Health and Care Excellence (NICE). Rivaroxaban for preventing atherothrombotic events in people with coronary or peripheral artery disease. 2019. https://www.nice.org.uk/guidance/ta607
6. COMPASS Investigators. Rivaroxaban with or without aspirin in patients with stable peripheral or carotid artery disease: An international, randomised, double-blind, placebo-controlled trial. *Lancet.* 2018;391(10117):219–229.

4

UK Medical Research Council/British Heart Foundation Heart Protection Study of Cholesterol Lowering with Simvastatin in 20,536 High-Risk Individuals

A Randomized Placebo-Controlled Trial

> Lowering LDL cholesterol with a statin produces a substantial reduction in the incidence of major vascular events.
>
> THE HEART PROTECTION STUDY INVESTIGATORS

Research Question: In patients with high risk for cardiovascular disease, does simvastatin reduce cardiovascular morbidity and mortality, as compared to placebo?[1]

Funding: UK Medical Research Council, the British Heart Foundation, Merck & Co. (manufacturers of simvastatin), and Roche Vitamins Ltd.

Year Study Began: 1994

Year Study Published: 2002

Study Location: 69 clinical centers from the UK

Who Was Studied: Patients 40–80 years of age were eligible provided they were considered to be at a substantial 5-year risk of death from coronary heart disease due to:

- Coronary disease (i.e., history of myocardial infarction [MI], unstable or stable angina, coronary artery bypass graft, or angioplasty)
- Non-disabling ischemic stroke, transient cerebral ischemia, or carotid endarterectomy
- Peripheral arterial disease (PAD; history of intermittent claudication, arterial surgery, or angioplasty)
- Diabetes mellitus (type 1 or type 2)
- Hypertension (if male and aged >65 years)

Who Was Excluded: Patients were excluded from the study if they had any of the following:

- Cholesterol <3.5 mmol/L
- Chronic liver disease
- Severe renal disease
- Severe heart failure
- Inflammatory muscle disease such as polymyositis
- Concurrent treatment with ciclosporin, fibrates, or high-dose niacin
- Life-threatening condition such as severe chronic airways disease or cancer

Patients: 20,536

Study Overview

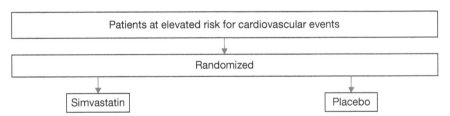

Figure 4.1 Design of Heart Protection randomized controlled trial

Study Intervention: Potentially eligible people entered a pre-randomization run-in phase to ensure that patients randomized would be compliant with study treatment. After the run-in, eligible patients were randomly assigned to receive 40 mg atorvastatin once a day or placebo once a day.

Follow-up: Mean duration of 5 years

Endpoints: The main outcome measures were mortality (all-cause and vascular) and major vascular events (coronary event, stroke, and revascularization).

RESULTS

- Of those who entered the run-in phase, 36% were not subsequently randomized, mainly due to patient choice/compliance (26%) or due to clear indication for statin use (5%).
- In the simvastatin group, average statin use during the scheduled treatment period was 85%, compared to 17% in the placebo group.
- All-cause mortality was significantly reduced in the allocated simvastatin group (12.9%) compared to the allocated placebo group (14.7%). Similarly, coronary death rate was significantly reduced (5.7% vs. 6.9%).
- Any major vascular event was significantly reduced in the allocated simvastatin group compared to the placebo group (19.8% vs. 25.2%).
- Reduction in major vascular event was found to be present in all subgroup analyses, including age, gender, cholesterol level, and smoking status, and during the entire period of follow-up (Table 4.1).
- Simvastatin was also found to have a safe profile with no differences found in terms of myalgia, cancer incidence, or treatment stopped due to elevated liver enzymes.

Table 4.1 EFFECTS OF SIMVASTATIN ALLOCATION ON FIRST MAJOR VASCULAR EVENT DURING FOLLOW-UP

Year of follow-up	Simvastatin	Placebo
1	481/10,269 (4.7%)	527/10,267 (5.1%)
2	377/9,745 (3.9%)	538/9,683 (5.6%)
3	359/9,288 (3.9%)	509/9,055 (5.6%)
4	331/8,818 (3.8%)	436/8,463 (5.2%)
5+	485/8,358 (5.8%)	575/7,897 (7.3%)
All follow-up	2033/10,269 (19.8%)	2585/10,267 (25.2%)

Criticisms and Limitations: Exclusion of participants after a run-in period due to adherence issues raises the possibility of selection bias, and therefore results may not be generalizable to real-world clinical practice.

Other Relevant Studies and Information: Mondillo et al. showed in their randomized controlled trial that simvastatin improved walking performance, ankle–brachial pressure indexes, and symptoms of claudication in hypercholesterolemic patients with PAD.[2] Similarly, Mohler at al. showed in a randomized controlled trial that patients treated with atorvastatin had greater pain-free walking distance than those receiving placebo.[3]

The Cholesterol Treatment Trialists' Collaboration published in 2010 a meta-analysis of data from 170,000 patients. They compared more intensive statin therapy and showed that it safely produced further reductions in the incidence of MI, revascularization, and ischemic stroke.[4]

The Global Vascular Guidelines on the management of chronic limb-threatening ischemia (CLTI) recommend the use of moderate- or high-intensity statin therapy to reduce all-cause and cardiovascular mortality in patients with CLTI.[5]

Summary and Implications: In patients with high risk for cardiovascular disease, simvastatin use is associated with a reduction in all-cause mortality and major vascular event risks, as compared to placebo. The benefit of cholesterol lowering was neither limited by a threshold LDL-C level nor dependent on the pretreatment cholesterol level. Patients with vascular disease without contraindications should be offered a statin.

CLINICAL CASE: CHOLESTEROL THERAPY FOR PAD

Case History
A 65-year-old woman with a history of intermittent claudication and angina attends your outpatient clinic. She would like advice on the best management of her cardiovascular risk. She is currently taking aspirin and amlodipine. Her cholesterol level is normal.

Suggested Answer
The Heart Protection Study trial showed a risk reduction in both all-cause mortality and coronary death in high-risk patients. This patient has a history of both coronary and peripheral artery disease and should be started on a high-dose statin. You explain to her that even though her cholesterol is within normal limits, she will still benefit from a statin.

References

1. Heart Protection Study Collaborative Group Writers. MRC/BHF Heart Protection Study of cholesterol lowering with simvastatin in 20,536 high-risk individuals: A randomised placebo-controlled trial. *Lancet.* 2002;360(9326):7–22.
2. Mondillo S, Ballo P, Barbati R, et al. Effects of simvastatin on walking performance and symptoms of intermittent claudication in hypercholesterolemic patients with peripheral vascular disease. *Am J Med.* 2003;114(5):359–364.
3. Mohler ER 3rd, Hiatt WR, Creager MA. Cholesterol reduction with atorvastatin improves walking distance in patients with peripheral arterial disease. *Circulation.* 2003;108(12):1481–1486.
4. Cholesterol Treatment Trialists' (CTT) Collaboration. Efficacy and safety of more intensive lowering of LDL cholesterol: A meta-analysis of data from 170,000 participants in 26 randomised trials *Lancet.* 2010;376(9753):1670–1681.
5. GVG Writing Group for the Joint Guidelines of the Society for Vascular Surgery (SVS), European Society for Vascular Surgery (ESVS), and World Federation of Vascular Societies (WFVS). Global vascular guidelines on the management of chronic limb-threatening ischemia. *Eur J Vasc Endovasc Surg.* 2019;58(1S):S1–S109.

5

Systematic Review of the Efficacy of Cilostazol, Naftidrofuryl Oxalate, and Pentoxifylline for the Treatment of Intermittent Claudication

> Naftidrofuryl oxalate and cilostazol are both effective treatments for claudication.
>
> STEVENS ET AL.

Research Question: Does cilostazol, naftidrofuryl oxalate, or pentoxifylline provide symptomatic relief for patients suffering from intermittent claudication?[1]

Funding: National Institute of Health Research Health Technology Assessment Programme

Year Range for Searches: 1963–2010

Year Study Published: 2012

Number of Studies Included in Systematic Review: 26 studies included in the systematic review with 11 randomized clinical trials included in the meta-analysis

Which Studies Were Included: A systematic review was conducted to identify the clinical effectiveness and adverse events of cilostazol, naftidrofuryl oxalate, pentoxifylline, and inositol nicotinate for the treatment of intermittent claudication in people with peripheral arterial disease (PAD). To be eligible for inclusion, studies had to be randomized controlled trials (RCTs) or systematic reviews, provided that they contained additional data not available in published study reports.

Which Studies Were Excluded: Studies were excluded if they were editorials, opinion pieces, reports published as meeting abstracts only, studies with those drugs not used within their licensed indications, studies in which the population was not restricted to Fontaine stage II, and studies that did not contain data for the included outcomes.

Study Overview: This was a systematic review and meta-analysis on the efficacy of cilostazol, naftidrofuryl oxalate, and pentoxifylline for the treatment of intermittent claudication. A comprehensive search strategy was used to include terms for intermittent claudication and peripheral arterial disease.

Follow-up: 24 weeks or more

Endpoints: *Primary outcomes:* Maximum walking distance (MWD) and pain-free walking distance (PFWD) at baseline and at the end of the study (at least 24 weeks of follow-up). *Secondary outcomes:* Adverse events and quality of life.

RESULTS

- Of the trials included in the meta-analysis, eight of the studies were conducted in the US, one was conducted in France, one in Sweden/ Denmark, and one in the UK.
- The meta-analysis reported results from six studies for cilostazol, six studies for pentoxifylline, and two studies for naftidrofuryl oxalate. Because there were no suitable studies on inositol nicotinate, it was excluded from the meta-analysis.
- All three treatments were associated with improvement in both MWD and PFWD when compared to placebo (Table 5.1).
- For naftidrofuryl oxalate, cilostazol, and pentoxifylline, MWD increased by 60%, 25%, and 11% respectively relative to placebo, and PFWD increased by 49%, 13%, and 9% respectively.
- The systematic review suggested that adverse events were generally minor and included headaches and gastrointestinal difficulties. The incidence of serious adverse events was reported to be low too.

- Quality-of-life scores were not reported in the studies included in the systematic review.

Table 5.1 PERCENTAGE CHANGE FROM BASELINE MWD AND PFWD COMPARED
WITH PLACEBO

Treatment	MWD (95% CI)	PFWD
Cilostazol	25 (11–40)	13 (2–26)
Naftidrofuryl oxalate	60 (20–114)	49 (23–81)
Pentoxifylline	11 (−1 to 24)	9 (−2 to 22)

CI, confidence interval.

Criticisms and Limitations

- MWD and PFWD may not be the ideal outcome measures. They do not necessarily correlate with quality-of-life improvements, which is the aim of any therapy for intermittent claudication. None of the studies included in the systematic review included data on quality of life.
- Investigators in the various RCTs do not follow a common protocol for assessing MWD, which will have contributed to heterogeneity between studies in the estimates of treatment effect.
- Studies generally involved short-term follow-up, with no study lasting beyond 24 weeks other than for cilostazol.

Other Relevant Studies and Information

- National Institute for Health and Care Excellence (NICE) guidelines state that naftidrofuryl oxalate is recommended as an option for the treatment of intermittent claudication in people with PAD for whom vasodilator therapy is considered appropriate after taking into account other treatment options.[2]
- On the other hand, 2016 the American Heart Association (AHA)/ American College of Cardiology (ACC) guideline on the management of patients with lower-extremity peripheral artery disease states that cilostazol is an effective medical therapy for treatment of leg symptoms and walking impairment due to claudication.[3]
- Global Vascular Guidelines on the management of chronic limb-threatening ischemia (CLTI) state that in the absence of RCTs in

patients with CLTI, there is insufficient evidence that cilostazol, naftidrofuryl oxalate, or pentoxifylline improves clinical outcomes in patients with CLTI.[4]

Summary and Implications: This systematic review has shown that naftidrofuryl oxalate and cilostazol are both effective treatments for claudication with respect to the outcomes of MWD and PFWD. Naftidrofuryl oxalate might be the more effective medication, but more evidence is available for the use of cilostazol.

CLINICAL CASE: MEDICATIONS FOR INTERMITTENT CLAUDICATION

Case History

A 63-year-old man attends clinic with a 100-yard claudication history. He is currently taking aspirin and simvastatin but he smokes 10 cigarettes a day. He works long hours as a shopkeeper, Monday to Saturday. On Sundays, he likes to walk around the local park with his grandchildren, but the claudication is restricting him. He tells you that the claudication has impaired his lifestyle and would like to know if there is any treatment he could have to improve his symptoms.

Suggested Answer

The COMPASS trial (see Chapter 2) has shown that if the patient has a low risk of bleeding and does not have any other contraindication, he would benefit from low-dose rivaroxaban in addition to his aspirin. He should be recommended to stop smoking immediately to reduce major adverse limb and cardiovascular events. Due to his work commitments, he is unable to regularly attend exercise classes. From the systematic review, he could be offered naftidrofuryl oxalate or cilostazol to improve his walking distance.

References

1. Stevens JW, Simpson E, Harnan S, et al. Systematic review of the efficacy of cilostazol, naftidrofuryl oxalate and pentoxifylline for the treatment of intermittent claudication. *Br J Surg.* 2012;99(12):1630–1638.
2. National Institute for Health and Care Excellence (NICE). Cilostazol, naftidrofuryl oxalate, pentoxifylline and inositol nicotinate for the treatment of intermittent

claudication in people with peripheral arterial disease. 2011. https://www.nice.org. uk/guidance/ta223

3. Gerhard-Herman MD, Gornik HL, Barrett C, et al. 2016 AHA/ACC guideline on the management of patients with lower extremity peripheral artery disease: A report of the American College of Cardiology/American Heart Association Task Force on Clinical Practice Guidelines. *Circulation.* 2017;135(12):e726–e779.

4. GVG Writing Group for the Joint Guidelines of the Society for Vascular Surgery (SVS), European Society for Vascular Surgery (ESVS), and World Federation of Vascular Societies (WFVS). Global vascular guidelines on the management of chronic limb-threatening ischemia. *Eur J Vasc Endovasc Surg.* 2019;58(1S):S1–S109.

Cerebrovascular Disease

JULIEN AL SHAKARCHI AND ALOK TIWARI

6

Analysis of Pooled Data from the Randomized Controlled Trials of Endarterectomy for Symptomatic Carotid Stenosis

> Surgery is of some benefit for patients with 50–69% symptomatic stenosis, and highly beneficial for those with 70% symptomatic stenosis or greater.
>
> ROTHWELL ET AL.

Research Question: Does carotid endarterectomy (CEA) reduce the risk of stroke in recently symptomatic patients with internal carotid artery (ICA) disease?[1]

Funding: Salaries from the first three authors were provided by the UK Stroke Association, UK Medical Research Council, and the National Institute of Neurological Disorders and Stroke.

Year Included Studies Were Published: European Carotid Surgery Trial (ECST, 1998), North American Symptomatic Carotid Endarterectomy Trial (NASCET, 1998), and Veterans Affairs 309 (VA309, 1991)

Year Study Published: 2003

Study Locations: ECST (100 centers in 14 European countries), NASCET (106 centers mainly in the US and Canada), and VA309 (16 centers in the US)

Who Was Studied: Adults who had (1) a recent carotid-distribution transient ischemic attack, non-disabling ischemic stroke, or a retinal infarction and (2) a stenosis of the ipsilateral ICA (imaged by angiography).

Who Was Excluded: Patients were excluded if symptoms had occurred >6 months ago, if the stroke was likely caused by cardiac embolus, if disease was more severe in the distal/intracranial ICA, or if the stroke was disabling.

Patients: 6,092

Study Overview

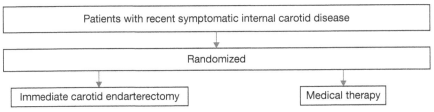

Figure 6.1 Design of randomized controlled trials

Study Intervention: The original individual patient data were obtained for the three trials. Data on presenting events, baseline clinical findings, imaging, surgical techniques, and follow-up were merged. Definitions were considered carefully to allow the data to be merged in this single database.

Follow-up: Mean duration of 65 months

Endpoints: Outcome measures were:
- Any stroke or operative death
- Ipsilateral ischemic stroke in the territory of the symptomatic carotid artery, and any stroke or death that occurred within 30 days of trial surgery
- Ipsilateral disabling or fatal ischemic stroke in the territory of the symptomatic carotid artery and any disabling stroke or death that occurred within 30 days of trial surgery

RESULTS

- Of the patients who were randomized to surgery, 3,248 (98%) out of 3,334 underwent trial surgery. The median time from randomization to trial surgery was 6 days.

- CEA decreased the 5-year risk of stroke or operative death in patients with 50–99% ICA stenosis. The greatest benefit was found in severe stenosis (70–99%). No benefit was found for patients with near occlusion or stenosis <50% (Table 6.1).
- Similar results were found for the 5-year risk of ipsilateral stoke and any operative stroke/death (see Table 6.1).
- The 5-year risk of an ipsilateral or fatal ischemic stroke and any operative disabling stoke/death was only reduced in patients with ICA stenosis of 70–99% (see Table 6.1).

Table 6.1 EFFECTS OF SURGERY ON MAIN STUDY OUTCOMES BY DEGREE OF SYMPTOMATIC CAROTID STENOSIS

Degree of ICA stenosis	5-year absolute risk reduction (95% CI): Any stroke or operative death	5-year absolute risk reduction (95% CI): Ipsilateral stroke and operative stroke or death	5-year absolute risk reduction (95% CI): Ipsilateral disabling or fatal stroke and operative disabling stroke or death
Near occlusion	−0.1% (−10.3 to 10.2)	−1.7% (−8.7 to 10.2)	−2.3% (−8.7 to 4.1)
70–99%	15.3% (9.8 to 20.7)	16.0% (11.2 to 20.8)	7.0% (3.6 to 10.4)
50–69%	7.8% (3.1 to 12.5)	4.6% (0.6 to 8.6)	2.3% (−0.3 to 4.8)
30–49%	2.6% (−1.7 to 6.9)	3.2% (−1.9 to 8.3)	0.5% (−2.3 to 3.3)
<30%	−2.6% (−6.2 to 0.9)	−2.2% (−6.0 to 1.6)	−1.7% (−3.5 to 0.3)

CI, confidence interval.

Criticisms and Limitations: Best medical therapy was not defined clearly in the studies. Aspirin was recommended at different doses and statins were not used routinely. Therefore, results might well be different if the trials were repeated in the modern era of best medical therapy. On the other hand, the delay to surgery was relatively long and the benefit of surgery might have been underestimated.

Other Relevant Studies and Information

- European Society for Vascular Surgery guidelines on the management of atherosclerotic carotid and vertebral artery disease recommend CEA in patients who have reported carotid territory symptoms within the preceding 6 months and who have a 70–99% carotid stenosis. The guidelines also recommend that patients with a 50–69% carotid stenosis should be considered for surgery.[2]

- The updated Society for Vascular Surgery guidelines for management of extracranial carotid disease recommend that patients with 50–99% carotid stenosis who are candidates for intervention should preferably have CEA.[3]
- The Clopidogrel with Aspirin in Acute Minor Stroke or Transient Ischemic Attack (CHANCE) trial showed a reduction in stroke rate with dual antiplatelet therapy in the first 90 days following a stroke or transient ischemic attack.[4]

Summary and Implications: The uncertain benefit of CEA for the secondary prevention of carotid artery territory stroke led to several major studies, including the ESCT and NASCET. This analysis of pooled data from the three main randomized controlled trials provides the strongest evidence for the benefit of CEA for patients with an ICA stenosis of 50–99%.

CLINICAL CASE: SYMPTOMATIC CAROTID ARTERY DISEASE

Case History

A 76-year-old man presents to the emergency department with left upper and lower limb weakness as well as facial drooping. A computed tomography (CT) scan reveals a right-sided ischemic stroke and his Rankin score is 2. The results of his cardiac investigations are normal and the duplex ultrasound reveals an 80% stenosis of his right ICA. How would you manage this patient?

Suggested Answer

This patient should be treated with dual antiplatelet therapy and high-intensity statin. In addition, his blood pressure should be well controlled. As per the pooled analysis, he should be offered a CEA to reduce his risk of future stroke. The surgery is carried out, and he makes a full recovery.

References

1. Rothwell PM, Eliasziw M, Gutnikov SA, et al. Analysis of pooled data from the randomised controlled trials of endarterectomy for symptomatic carotid stenosis. *Lancet.* 2003;361:107–116.
2. Naylor AR, Ricco JB, de Borst GJ, et al. Editor's choice—management of atherosclerotic carotid and vertebral artery disease: 2017 clinical practice guidelines

of the European Society for Vascular Surgery (ESVS). *Eur J Vasc Endovasc Surg.* 2018;55:3–81.

3. AbuRahma AF, Avgerinos ED, Chang RW, et al. The Society for Vascular Surgery implementation document for management of extracranial cerebrovascular disease. *J Vasc Surg.* 2022;75(1S):26S–98S.

4. CHANCE Investigators. Clopidogrel with Aspirin in Acute Minor Stroke or Transient Ischemic Attack (CHANCE) trial: One-year outcomes. *Circulation.* 2015;132(1):40–46.

7

Early Endarterectomy Carries a Lower Procedural Risk Than Early Stenting in Patients with Symptomatic Stenosis of the Internal Carotid Artery

> Risk differences between [carotid stenting] and [carotid endarterectomy] were greatest in the early days after the index symptom.
>
> RANTNER ET AL.

Research Question: Is carotid endarterectomy (CEA) safer than carotid stenting (CAS) in the early period following a stroke in patients with symptomatic stenosis of the internal carotid artery?[1]

Funding: No external funding

Year Study Published: 2017

Number of Studies Included: Four randomized clinical trials (Rcts): Endarterectomy Versus Angioplasty in Patients with Symptomatic Severe Carotid Stenosis (EVA-3S), Stent-Protected Angioplasty Versus Carotid Endarterectomy (SPACE), International Carotid Stenting Study (ICSS), and Carotid Revascularization Endarterectomy Versus Stenting Trial (CREST)

Who Was Studied: Patients were eligible to be included if they were deemed suitable to have either CEA or CAS and if:

- They had symptomatic moderate to severe carotid stenosis (≥50% North American Symptomatic Carotid Endarterectomy Trial [NASCET] criteria) for EVA-3S, SPACE, and ICSS.
- They had symptomatic carotid artery stenosis of ≥50% on invasive angiography, ≥70% on ultrasound, or ≥70% on computed tomographic or magnetic resonance angiography if the stenosis was 50–69% on ultrasound for CREST.

Who Was Excluded: Patients with recurrent stenosis, asymptomatic carotid artery disease, and limited life expectancy were excluded from the studies.

Patients: 4,138

Study Overview: This was a meta-analysis of data from four RCTs comparing CEA versus CAS for patients with symptomatic carotid artery disease. This analysis focused on the effects of procedural timing on outcomes.

Study Intervention: Pooled analysis of individual patient data from four RCTs. Patients were randomly assigned to CEA or CAS following a neurologic event.

Follow-up: This pooled analysis specifically looked at early 30-day outcomes.

Endpoints: *Primary outcome:* Composite of any stroke or death occurring within 30 days after treatment. *Secondary outcomes:* Any stroke and fatal or disabling stroke happening within 30 days after treatment.

RESULTS

- The median delay between the most recent neurologic event and treatment was 26 days (interquartile range [IQR]: 11–61) for CAS and 29 days (IQR: 13–67) for CEA. Among 4,138 patients, a small but relevant group (n = 513) underwent CAS and CEA within a week of their symptoms (14% in CAS vs. 11% in CEA) (Table 7.1).
- The risk of any stroke or death within 30 days after treatment was higher for the CAS compared with the CEA group for the entire study population: 7.3% versus 3.3% (crude relative risk [RR] = 2.29; 95% confidence interval (CI): 1.71–3.08).
- In the early period after the onset of neurologic symptoms (0–7 days), CAS had the highest number and proportion of periprocedural strokes

and deaths (n = 24/287, 8.4%), compared with CEA (n = 3/226, 1.3%). Patients in the CAS group had a higher risk of any stroke or death (RR = 6.51; 95% CI: 2.00–21.21).

- Compared with those treated within 7 days, patients treated after 7 days had fewer strokes and deaths in the CAS group (n = 129/1806, 7.1%), whereas the risk of stroke and death in the CEA group slightly increased (n = 65/1819, 3.6%). The risk for CAS compared with CEA was still higher in this later treatment group (RR = 2.00; 95% CI: 1.49–2.67).

Table 7.1 Outcomes within 30 days after treatment depending on timing of treatment

	Carotid endarterectomy	Carotid artery stenting	Crude RR	p value
Any stroke or death				
0–7 days	3/226 (1.3%)	24/287 (8.4%)	6.51	0.002
>7 days	65/1,819 (3.6%)	129/1,806 (7.1%)	2.00	<0.0001
Any stroke				
0–7 days	3/226 (1.3%)	23/287 (8.0%)	6.27	0.002
>7 days	62/1,819 (3.4%)	122/1,806 (6.8%)	1.98	<0.0001
Fatal or disabling stroke				
0–7 days	1/226 (0.4%)	9/287 (3.1%)	8.29	0.04
>7 days	26/1,819 (1.4%)	46/1,806 (2.5%)	1.77	0.02

Criticisms and Limitations

- Timing of treatment has to date never been a randomization criterion in larger trials. All information on the influence of timing of treatment is derived from post hoc analysis of RCTs. Therefore, detailed information on patient selection and disease severity is lacking. This significantly limits the value of timing analysis to date; thus, a randomized trial on timing of treatment is required for firm conclusions.
- The use of embolic protection devices was mandatory in the CREST trial but not in the other three trials. Therefore, the results for CAS might have been different if these devices were used in all patients.
- Transcarotid artery revascularization (TCAR) was not investigated in any of the trials.

Other Relevant Studies and Information

- According to the recently published carotid guidelines from the Society for Vascular Surgery, CEA is preferred over transfemoral CAS in symptomatic patients with ≥50% stenosis who are candidates for both procedures. TCAR is preferred over transfemoral CAS but not CEA in symptomatic patients with ≥50% stenosis.[2]
- The European Society for Vascular Surgery guidelines recommend that most patients who have suffered carotid territory symptoms within the preceding 6 months and who are aged >70 years and who have 50–99% stenoses should be treated by CEA rather than carotid stenting.[3]

Summary and Implications: In the early period following the onset of symptomatic carotid artery stenosis, CEA is associated with considerably lower periprocedural complication rates than CAS.

CLINICAL CASE: STENTING FOR SYMPTOMATIC CAROTID ARTERY DISEASE

Case History

A 79-year-old woman presents to the emergency department with right upper and lower limb weakness. A computed tomography scan reveals a right-sided ischemic stroke and her Rankin score is 2. Her cardiac investigations are normal and the duplex ultrasound reveals a 90% stenosis of her right internal carotid artery. The patient has been told that she could have keyhole surgery. How would you manage this patient?

Suggested Answer

This patient should be treated with dual antiplatelet therapy and high-intensity statin. In addition, her blood pressure should be well controlled. As per the pooled analysis, she should be offered a CEA to reduce her risk of future stroke. She should be advised that the evidence suggests that open surgery offers a higher stroke-prevention benefit. She accepts your advice and makes a full recovery following a CEA.

References

1. Rantner B, Kollerits B, Roubin GS, et al. Early endarterectomy carries a lower procedural risk than early stenting in patients with symptomatic stenosis of the internal carotid artery. *Stroke.* 2017;48(6):1580–1587.
2. AbuRahma AF, Avgerinos ED, Chang RW, et al. The Society for Vascular Surgery implementation document for management of extracranial cerebrovascular disease. *J Vasc Surg.* 2022;75(1S):26S–98S.
3. Naylor AR, Ricco JB, de Borst GJ, et al. Editor's choice—management of atherosclerotic carotid and vertebral artery disease: 2017 clinical practice guidelines of the European Society for Vascular Surgery (ESVS). *Eur J Vasc Endovasc Surg.* 2018;55:3–81.

8

Prevention of Disabling and Fatal Strokes by Successful Carotid Endarterectomy in Patients Without Recent Neurologic Symptoms

First Asymptomatic Carotid Surgery Trial (ACST-1), a Randomized Controlled Trial

> Among [asymptomatic] patients . . . with severe carotid stenosis . . . [carotid endarterectomy] approximately halved the net 5-year risk of stroke . . . [However,] the balance of risk and benefit depends on surgical morbidity rates . . . and on the risk of carotid stroke in the absence of surgery.
>
> THE ACST-1 INVESTIGATORS

Research Question: Is carotid endarterectomy (CEA) beneficial in asymptomatic patients with carotid artery disease?[1]

Funding: The United Kingdom Medical Research Council and the Stroke Association

Year Study Began: 1993

Year Study Published: 2004

Study Location: 126 clinical centers from 30 countries

Who Was Studied: Patients were included in the study if:
- They had severe unilateral or bilateral carotid artery stenosis
- The stenosis had not caused stroke, transient cerebral ischemia, or any other relevant neurologic symptoms in the past 6 months
- No circumstance or condition precluded long-term follow-up

Who Was Excluded: Patients with a prior ipsilateral CEA, patients at high surgical risk, and patients with other major medical problems. In addition, surgeons with high complication rates (>6% rates of perioperative stroke or death) were not eligible to participate in the trial.

Patients: 3,120

Study Overview

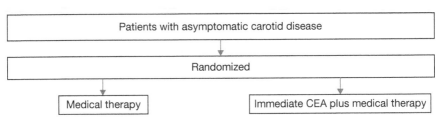

Figure 8.1 Design of ACST-1 randomized controlled trial

Study Intervention: Patients were randomly assigned to medical therapy or CEA. Patients in the CEA group were offered the procedure immediately. In contrast, patients in the medical therapy group only received surgery if they developed symptoms due to the stenosis, if a hard indication for CEA arose, or if the doctor or patient changed their mind. In both groups, patients received standard medical care for atherosclerotic disease.

Follow-up: Mean duration of 9 years

Endpoints: Primary outcome was perioperative mortality and morbidity (death or stroke within 30 days) and non-perioperative stroke.

RESULTS

- ~90% of patients in the CEA group underwent CEA within a year of enrollment versus ~5% of patients in the medical therapy group (typically due to the development of a hard indication for CEA) (Table 8.1).
- ~26% of patients in the medical therapy group underwent CEA within 10 years of enrollment, mostly due to the development of a hard indication for CEA. 2.9% of patients in the immediate CEA group experienced perioperative stroke or death, compared to 3.6% in the deferred CEA group.
- For the first 2 years of the trial, patients in the medical therapy group had better outcomes than those in the CEA group because of the high rate of perioperative strokes and death among patients assigned to CEA. However, after 2 years, the benefits of CEA became apparent.
- Both men and women ultimately benefited from CEA; however, patients age >75 at trial entry did not.

Table 8.1 PERIOPERATIVE MORTALITY AND MORBIDITY

	Immediate CEA group (n = 1,560)	Deferred CEA group (n = 1,560)
Total number of CEAs	1532	447
Stroke death	11	2
Cardiac death	5	0
Other death	1	1
Disabling stroke	9	5
Non-disabling stroke	18	8
Nonfatal myocardial infarction	10	1
Any perioperative stroke or death	44	16
% of total number of CEAs	2.9%	3.6%

Criticisms and Limitations: Since the time ACST was conducted, medical therapy for atherosclerotic disease has evolved. For example, at the beginning of the trial, only 17% of patients were taking lipid-lowering medications. It is possible that the benefits of CEA may be less pronounced now that medical therapies have improved.

In addition, surgeons with high complication rates were not invited to participate in the trial, and therefore it is possible that the benefits of CEA may be lower in "real-world settings" in which some CEAs are performed by less-skilled surgeons.

Other Relevant Studies and Information

- The Asymptomatic Carotid Atherosclerosis Study (ACAS) also evaluated CEA in asymptomatic patients and came to similar conclusions as the ACST trial. A meta-analysis involving data from ACAS and ACST raised questions about the effectiveness of CEA for asymptomatic carotid disease among women. This meta-analysis did not include long-term follow-up data from ACST, however.[2]
- The recently published Society for Vascular Surgery carotid guidelines state that neurologically asymptomatic patients with a stenosis diameter of ≥70% should be considered for CEA.[3]
- The European Society for Vascular Surgery recommends that in "average surgical risk" patients with an asymptomatic 60–99% stenosis, CEA should be considered in the presence of one or more imaging characteristics that may be associated with an increased risk of late ipsilateral stroke. These characteristics include silent infarction on computed tomography/ magnetic resonance imaging, stenosis progression, and large plaque area.[4]

Summary and Implications: In patients with asymptomatic carotid athero-sclerotic disease (stenosis ≥60%), CEA is associated with a perioperative risk of ~3%. After 2–3 years, patients who receive surgery have a lower rate of stroke than those treated medically. The decision about whether or not to proceed with surgery depends on patient preference, life expectancy, and the skill of the involved surgeon.

CLINICAL CASE: ASYMPTOMATIC CAROTID ARTERY DISEASE

Case History

A family doctor asks your expert opinion for a 65-year-old man with a history of intermittent claudication. The patient was found to have a carotid bruit and an ultrasound duplex has shown a 79% internal carotid artery stenosis. He is an ex-smoker and currently takes aspirin and atorvastatin. He would like advice on the management of the carotid artery disease.

Suggested Answer

The ACST study has shown that patients with asymptomatic carotid artery disease benefit in the long term from CEA. The patient should be offered the option of surgery but should be told that medical management has evolved since the trial and the benefit is now unclear.

References

1. Halliday A, Mansfield A, Marro J, et al. Prevention of disabling and fatal strokes by successful carotid endarterectomy in patients without recent neurological symptoms: Randomized controlled trial (ACST). *Lancet*. 2004;363(9420):1491–1502.
2. Rothwell PM, Goldstein LB. Carotid endarterectomy for asymptomatic carotid stenosis: Asymptomatic Carotid Surgery Trial. *Stroke*. 2004;35(10):2425–2427.
3. AbuRahma AF, Avgerinos ED, Chang RW, et al. The Society for Vascular Surgery implementation document for management of extracranial cerebrovascular disease. *J Vasc Surg*. 2022;75(1S):26S–98S.
4. Naylor AR, Ricco JB, de Borst GJ, et al. Editor's choice—management of atherosclerotic carotid and vertebral artery disease: 2017 clinical practice guidelines of the European Society for Vascular Surgery (ESVS). *Eur J Vasc Endovasc Surg*. 2018;55:3–81.

9

Safety of Stenting and Endarterectomy for Asymptomatic Carotid Artery Stenosis

A Meta-analysis of Randomized Controlled Trials

This study indicates that carotid endarterectomy has a lower rate of periprocedural stroke than carotid artery stenting.

CUI ET AL.

Research Question: Is carotid artery stenting (CAS) as safe as carotid endarterectomy (CEA) in asymptomatic patients with carotid artery disease?[1]

Funding: National Science Foundation of China

Year Range for Searches: 1963–2017

Year Study Published: 2018

Number of Studies Included: Five suitable randomized controlled trials (RCTs) were included in the meta-analysis.

Which Studies Were Included: To be eligible for inclusion, studies had to be an RCT comparing any peri- or post-procedural outcomes between CAS and CEA for asymptomatic adults with unilateral or bilateral carotid artery stenosis.

Which Studies Were Excluded: Observational or retrospective studies were excluded, as well as conference abstracts, editorials, and commentaries. RCTs published without respective outcomes of the two interventions were also excluded.

Patients: 3,901

Study Overview: A meta-analysis of RCTs was performed to evaluate the safety of CAS versus CEA for asymptomatic carotid stenosis. A comprehensive search strategy was used to include terms for carotid stenosis, stents, and carotid endarterectomy.

Follow-up: Range 4–10 years

Endpoints: Perioperative mortality, any perioperative stroke, ipsilateral perioperative stroke, and perioperative myocardial infarction (MI)

RESULTS

- The study found no significant difference in terms of the risk associated with periprocedural death (CAS: n = 1/1,229 [0.1%]; CEA: n = 1/505 [0.2%]; odds ratio [OR] 1.49, 95% confidence interval [CI] 0.26–8.68) (Table 9.1).
- The fixed-effects model revealed that endarterectomy tended to be associated with a lower rate of periprocedural stroke than stenting (CAS: n = 47/1,823 [2.6%]; CEA: n = 14/1,092 [1.3%]; OR 0.53; 95% CI 0.29–0.96).
- There was no significant difference between the incidence of periprocedural ipsilateral stroke (CAS: n = 27/1,229 [2.2%]; CEA: n = 6/505 [1.2%]; OR 0.63, 95% CI 0.27–1.47).
- No significant difference was found in the incidence of periprocedural MI (CAS: n = 12/1,823 [0.7%]; CEA: n = 16/1,092 [1.5%]; OR 1.75, 95% CI 0.84–3.65).
- Most trials reported that the mid- to long-term outcomes were similar between stenting and endarterectomy.

Table 9.1 PERIOPERATIVE MORTALITY AND MORBIDITY

Outcome	CEA	CAS	p value
Any stroke	14/1,092 (1.3%)	47/1,823 (2.6%)	0.037
Death	1/505 (0.2%)	1/1,229 (0.1%)	0.657
MI	16/1,092 (1.5%)	12/1,823 (0.7%)	0.136
Ipsilateral stroke	6/505 (1.2%)	27/1,229 (2.2%)	0.283

Criticisms and Limitations: This study has several limitations. It was restricted to a limited number of published RCTs that were available in online databases. Differences in study protocols and definitions of clinical outcomes used contributed to the heterogeneity among the studies. Deficiencies in consistent outcome definitions prevented these data from being pooled. No mid- to long-term evaluations or subgroup analysis could be conducted.

Other Relevant Studies and Information

- The 2021 Society for Vascular Surgery carotid guidelines state that neurologically asymptomatic patients with a stenosis diameter of ≥70% should be considered for CEA. The determination of which technique to use should be based on the presence or absence of high-risk criteria for CEA, transcarotid artery revascularization (TCAR), or transfemoral CAS.[2]
- The European Society for Vascular Surgery recommends that in "average surgical risk" patients with an asymptomatic 60–99% stenosis if they have high-risk characteristics such as silent infarction on computed tomography/magnetic resonance imaging, stenosis progression, and large plaque area.[3] Otherwise, medical management can be practiced for asymptomatic carotid artery disease.

Summary and Implications: The meta-analysis indicates that CEA is associated with more favorable periprocedural outcomes with respect to any stroke. Based on this finding, CEA is the preferred is first-line treatment for patients with asymptomatic carotid stenosis 60–99% who opt for a surgical intervention.

CLINICAL CASE: STENTING FOR ASYMPTOMATIC CAROTID ARTERY DISEASE

Case History

A family doctor asks your expert opinion for a 70-year-old man with a history of intermittent claudication. The patient was found to have a carotid bruit and an ultrasound duplex has shown an 80–90% internal carotid artery stenosis. He is on medical therapy with clopidogrel and atorvastatin. He has a past medical history of neck surgery for cancer. He would like advice on the management of the carotid artery disease.

Suggested Answer

The ACST-1 study has shown that patients with asymptomatic carotid artery disease benefit in the long term from CEA. However, this patient is at a higher surgical risk due to the history of neck surgery for cancer. Therefore, the patient should be offered the option of carotid stenting but should be told that medical management has evolved since the ACST-1 trial and the benefit is now unclear.

References

1. Cui L, Han Y, Zhang S, et al. Safety of stenting and endarterectomy for asymptomatic carotid artery stenosis: A meta-analysis of randomised controlled trials. *Eur J Vasc Endovasc Surg.* 2018;55(5):614–624.
2. AbuRahma AF, Avgerinos ED, Chang RW, et al. The Society for Vascular Surgery implementation document for management of extracranial cerebrovascular disease. *J Vasc Surg.* 2022;75(1S):26S–98S.
3. Naylor AR, Ricco JB, de Borst GJ, et al. Editor's choice—management of atherosclerotic carotid and vertebral artery disease: 2017 clinical practice guidelines of the European Society for Vascular Surgery (ESVS). *Eur J Vasc Endovasc Surg.* 2018;55:3–81.

10

Second Asymptomatic Carotid Surgery Trial (ACST-2)

A Randomized Comparison of Carotid Artery Stenting Versus Carotid Endarterectomy

The main finding from the ACST-2 trial of [carotid artery stenting] versus [carotid endarterectomy] is that the effects of the two procedures on disabling or fatal events are approximately equal. . . . Non-disabling procedural stroke rates appeared to be slightly higher with [carotid artery stenting].

THE ACST-2 INVESTIGATORS

Research Question: What are the long-term results of carotid endarterectomy (CEA) versus carotid artery stenting (CAS) for asymptomatic patients with carotid artery disease?[1]

Funding: UK Medical Research Council and Health Technology Assessment Programme

Year Study Began: 2008

Year Study Published: 2021

Study Location: 130 clinical centers from 33 countries

Who Was Studied: Patients were included in the study if:

1. They had severe unilateral or bilateral carotid artery stenosis (>60%)
2. The stenosis had not caused stroke, transient cerebral ischemia, or any other relevant neurologic symptoms in the past 6 months
3. Computed tomography or magnetic resonance imaging confirmed suitability for CAS and for CEA
4. No circumstance or condition precluded long-term follow-up

Who Was Excluded: Exclusion criteria were previous ipsilateral intervention, unsuitability for CAS (due to calcification or tortuosity) or CEA, high procedural risk (e.g., due to recent acute myocardial infarction [MI]), high risk of cardiac emboli, or any major life-threatening condition.

Patients: 3,625

Study Overview

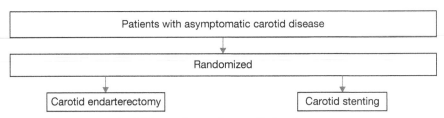

Figure 10.1 Design of ACST-2 randomized controlled trial

Study Intervention: Randomized controlled trial in which patients were randomly assigned to CEA or CAS.

Follow-up: Mean duration of 4.9 years

Endpoints: Study outcomes were procedural mortality and morbidity (i.e., onset before 30 days after the intervention) and non-procedural stroke, subdivided by severity.

RESULTS

- Among those allocated to CAS, 1,578 (87%) had it within 1 year, at a median of 14 days (interquartile range [IQR] 4–33) after randomization; 101 (6%) crossed over to CEA; and 106 (6%) had no intervention.

Among those allocated to CEA, 1,668 (92%) had it within 1 year, again at a median of 14 days (IQR 4–33) after randomization; 48 (3%) crossed over to CAS; and 78 (4%) had no intervention (Table 10.1).

- The risk of periprocedural stroke was higher in the CAS group (3.6%) compared to the CEA group, whereas the risk of periprocedural MI was higher following CEA (0.7%) than CAS (0.2%).
- Kaplan–Meier estimates of 5-year non-procedural stroke were 2.5% in each group for fatal or disabling stroke, and 5.3% with CAS versus 4.5% with CEA for any stroke (rate ratio [RR] 1.16, 95% confidence interval 0.86–1.57; p = 0.33).
- Subgroup analyses showed no significant difference in outcomes for age, sex, stenosis, plaque echolucency, and contralateral stenosis.

Table 10.1 DEATH, STROKE, OR MI WITHIN 30 DAYS OF
FIRST CAROTID PROCEDURE

	Allocated CAS (n = 1,811)	Allocated CEA (n = 1,814)	p value
Had a carotid procedure	1,705	1,736	
Any stroke	61 (3.6%)	41 (2.4%)	0.06
Any MI	5 (0.3%)	12 (0.7%)	0.15
Other death	2	2	1
Death, MI, or any stroke	67 (3.9%)	55 (3.2%)	0.26
Death or stroke	63 (3.7%)	47 (2.7%)	0.12

Criticisms and Limitations: One of the limitations of ACST-2 is the study size; although it is the largest carotid intervention trial yet conducted, the event rate was low in both groups. Therefore, the trial results must still be considered together with all other trials of CAS versus CEA.

A major criticism of the trial is a lack of a medical arm for asymptomatic patients. There is strong belief among a significant number of clinicians that modern medical management for asymptomatic patients is as good as an invasive intervention. Therefore, a third arm in the trial would have helped in this debate.

Other Relevant Studies and Information

- Both the Asymptomatic Carotid Atherosclerosis Study (ACAS) and the first ACST study (see Chapter 8) had previously shown a benefit for CEA in asymptomatic patients compared to medical treatment.[2,3]

- The Stent-Protected Angioplasty Versus Carotid Endarterectomy (SPACE-2) trial, which was stopped early due to poor recruitment (513 patients), showed no significant difference in 1-year outcome between surgery, stenting, and best medical therapy.[4]
- The recently published Society for Vascular Surgery carotid guidelines state that neurologically asymptomatic patients with a stenosis diameter of ≥70% should be considered for CEA, transcarotid artery revascularization (TCAR), or transfemoral CAS.[5]
- The European Society for Vascular Surgery recommends that in "average surgical risk" patients with an asymptomatic 60–99% stenosis, carotid stenting may be an alternative to CEA if the documented risk of stroke/death is <3%.[6]

Summary and Implications: Serious complications are similarly uncommon after competent CAS and CEA, and the long-term effects of these two carotid artery procedures on fatal or disabling stroke are comparable.

CLINICAL CASE: ASYMPTOMATIC CAROTID ARTERY DISEASE

Case History
A family doctor asks your expert opinion for a 65-year-old man with a history of ischemic heart disease with two previous MIs. The patient was found to have a carotid bruit and an ultrasound duplex has shown a 70–80% internal carotid artery stenosis. He is an ex-smoker and currently takes aspirin and atorvastatin. He would like advice on the carotid artery disease with a view to intervention.

Suggested Answer
The ACST-1 study showed that patients with asymptomatic carotid artery disease benefit in the long term from carotid intervention. The ACST-2 study has provided evidence that both CAS and CEA are safe options with comparable long-term results. In view of his cardiac risk, the patient decided to opt for CAS, although he is aware of the slightly increased risk of stroke.

References

1. Halliday A, Bulbulia R, Bonati LH, et al. Second asymptomatic carotid surgery trial (ACST-2): A randomised comparison of carotid artery stenting versus carotid endarterectomy. *Lancet.* 2021;398(10305):1065–1073.

2. Halliday A, Mansfield A, Marro J, et al. Prevention of disabling and fatal strokes by successful carotid endarterectomy in patients without recent neurological symptoms: Randomized controlled trial (ACST). *Lancet.* 2004;363(9420):1491–1502.
3. Walker MD, Marler JR, Goldstein M, et al. Endarterectomy for asymptomatic carotid artery stenosis. *JAMA.* 1995;273(18):1421–1428.
4. Reiff T, Eckstein HH, Mansmann U, et al. Angioplasty in asymptomatic carotid artery stenosis vs. endarterectomy compared to best medical treatment: One-year interim results of SPACE-2. *Int J Stroke.* 2019;15(6):1747493019833017.
5. AbuRahma AF, Avgerinos ED, Chang RW, et al. The Society for Vascular Surgery implementation document for management of extracranial cerebrovascular disease. *J Vasc Surg.* 2022;75(1S):26S–98S.
6. Naylor AR, Ricco JB, de Borst GJ, et al. Editor's choice—management of atherosclerotic carotid and vertebral artery disease: 2017 clinical practice guidelines of the European Society for Vascular Surgery (ESVS). *Eur J Vasc Endovasc Surg.* 2018;55:3–81.

11

General Anesthesia Versus Local Anesthesia for Carotid Surgery (GALA)

A Multicenter, Randomized Controlled Trial

There is no reason to prefer general over local anesthesia, or vice versa.

THE GALA INVESTIGATORS

Research Question: Which type of anesthesia is safer for patients undergoing carotid endarterectomy (CEA)?[1]

Funding: The Health Foundation (UK) and European Society of Vascular Surgery

Year Study Began: 1999

Year Study Published: 2008

Study Location: 95 clinical centers from 24 countries

Who Was Studied: Patients with symptomatic or asymptomatic internal carotid stenosis, for whom open surgery with either local or general anesthesia was advised, were eligible.

Who Was Excluded: Exclusion criteria included a simultaneous bilateral CEA; CEA combined with another operative procedure such as coronary artery bypass surgery; or if patients had previously taken part in the trial.

Patients: 3,526

Study Overview

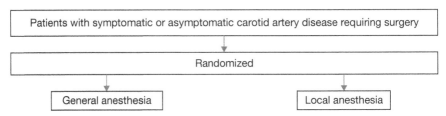

Figure 11.1 Design of GALA randomized controlled trial

Study Intervention: This was a two-arm, parallel-group, multicenter study of general anesthesia versus local anesthesia for carotid surgery.

Follow-up: Median follow-up 1 year

Endpoints: *Primary outcome:* Proportion of patients with stroke (including retinal infarction), myocardial infarction (MI), or death within 30 days of anesthesia (or 30 days after randomization for the few patients who did not have surgery). *Secondary outcomes:* Survival free of stroke, MI, or death up to 1 year after anesthesia; length of stay in recovery, high-dependency units, intensive-therapy units, and overall in hospital and health-related quality of life at about 30 days after anesthesia.

RESULTS

- Primary outcomes arose in 84 of 1,752 (4.8%) patients allocated to general anesthesia and 80 of 1,771 (4.5%) patients allocated to local anesthesia; the rate was not significantly different (Table 11.1).
- Time to first stroke, MI, or death at 1 year did not differ significantly between the two groups.
- There were no significant differences in any of the timing-related outcomes and no substantial difference for quality of life at ~30 days.
- The effect of general and local anesthesia on the primary outcome was not significantly different in the three prespecified subgroups (age, surgical risk, and contralateral carotid occlusion) or the post-hoc subgroups (trainee surgeon, trainee anesthetist, country, and asymptomatic stenosis).

Table 11.1 Perioperative mortality and morbidity

	General anesthesia (n = 1,753)	Local anesthesia (n = 1,773)	Risk ratio
Stroke, MI, or death	84 (4.8%)	80 (4.5%)	0.94 (95% CI 0.70–1.27)
Stroke	70 (4%)	66 (3.7%)	0.93 (95% CI 0.67–1.30
MI	4 (0.2%)	9 (0.5%)	
Other vascular death	9 (0.5%)	5 (0.3%)	
Death (any cause)	26 (1.5%)	19 (1.1%)	0.72 (95% CI 0.40–1.30)

CI, confidence interval.

Criticisms and Limitations: The stroke and death rates following CEA were low, which meant it was unlikely that the GALA trial would show any significant difference between local and general anesthesia, especially as they did not meet the recruitment target (5,000 patients).

Medication use such as preoperative statin use was not recorded; this might have mediated the impact of anesthesia choice on the risk of perioperative stroke.

Finally, intraoperative shunt usage rates varied considerably between the two groups (43% vs. 14%, for general vs. local anesthesia, respectively; $p < 0.0001$), as well as between UK and non-UK surgeons who always (73.6% vs. 20.8%, respectively; $p < 0.0001$), never (4.2% vs. 26%, respectively; $p < 0.0002$), or selectively (22.2% vs. 53.2%, respectively; $p < 0.0001$) used a shunt. Similarly, the use of patch was not standardized. These surgical confounding factors could well have implications on the risk of perioperative stroke.

Other Relevant Studies and Information

- The recently published Society for Vascular Surgery carotid guidelines state that the choice of local/regional versus general anesthesia should be left to the surgeon's/anesthesiologist's preference because both techniques have similar outcomes and should be based on availability of expertise for effective block.[2]
- Similarly, the European Society for Vascular Surgery recommends that choice of anesthesia for CEA (general vs. locoregional) should be left to the surgical team's discretion.[3]
- A Cochrane review published in 2013 found that the proportion of patients who had a stroke or died within 30 days of surgery did not differ significantly between the two types of anesthetic techniques

used during CEA. This systematic review provides evidence to suggest that patients and surgeons can choose either anesthetic technique, depending on the clinical situation and their own preferences.[4]

Summary and Implications: The GALA trial did not show a significant difference in outcomes between general and local anesthesia for carotid surgery. The anesthetist and surgeon, in consultation with the patient, should decide which anesthetic technique to use on an individual basis.

CLINICAL CASE: ANESTHESIA FOR CEA

Case History
A 79-year-old man suffers a right-sided ischemic stroke and makes a good recovery from it. An ultrasound duplex reveals a severe stenosis (80–89%) of the right internal carotid artery by an atherosclerotic plaque. A CEA is scheduled. The patient asks if he will be awake during the procedure.

Suggested Answer
You explain to the patient that there is no evidence of any difference in outcome between regional and general anesthesia. It is a decision to be made by the anesthetist, surgeon, and patient. He tells you that he is very anxious about the surgery and would prefer general anesthesia. The anesthetist is happy to proceed with this and the CEA is carried out without any complications. The patient makes a full recovery.

References

1. Lewis SC, Warlow CP, Bodenham AR, et al. General anaesthesia versus local anaesthesia for carotid surgery (GALA): A multicentre, randomised controlled trial. *Lancet.* 2008;372:2132–2142.
2. AbuRahma AF, Avgerinos ED, Chang RW, et al. The Society for Vascular Surgery implementation document for management of extracranial cerebrovascular disease *J Vasc Surg.* 2022;75(1S):26S–98S.
3. Naylor AR, Ricco JB, de Borst GJ, et al. Editor's choice—management of atherosclerotic carotid and vertebral artery disease: 2017 clinical practice guidelines of the European Society for Vascular Surgery (ESVS). *Eur J Vasc Endovasc Surg.* 2018;55:3–81.
4. Vaniyapong T, Chongruksut W, Rerkasem K. Local versus general anaesthesia for carotid endarterectomy. *Cochrane Database Syst Rev.* 2013;12:CD000126.

12

Prospective Randomized Trial of Carotid Endarterectomy with Primary Closure and Patch Angioplasty with Saphenous Vein, Jugular Vein, and Polytetrafluoroethylene

Long-Term Follow-up

Patching in general is superior to [primary closure] in lowering the incidence of perioperative stroke [during carotid endarterectomy].

ABURAHMA ET AL.

Research Question: Does patch closure provide a benefit compared to primary closure during carotid endarterectomy (CEA)?[1]

Funding: No external funding

Year Study Began: 1991

Year Study Published: 1998

Study Location: Single clinical center from the US

Who Was Studied: Adult patients who had asymptomatic or symptomatic carotid artery disease and who were scheduled for a CEA were eligible for inclusion.

Who Was Excluded: Patients who were scheduled for a repeat CEA or for CEA with concomitant coronary artery bypass grafting, or patients who had an internal carotid artery diameter <4 mm were excluded.

Patients: 399

Study Overview

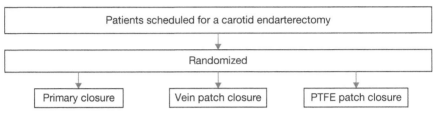

Figure 12.1 Design of randomized controlled trial

Study Intervention: Patients were randomly assigned to primary closure, vein patch closure or polytetrafluoroethylene (PTFE) patch closure. In the vein patch closure group, both saphenous veins at the ankle and jugular veins were used. All surgeries were performed with patients under general anesthesia and with routine shunting.

Follow-up: Mean duration of 30 months

Endpoints: Early outcomes were death, transient ischemic attacks (TIA), reversible ischemic neurologic deficits (RIND), and stroke. Long-term outcomes included recurrent stenosis and stroke-free survival.

RESULTS

- Early ipsilateral strokes were statistically significantly higher in patients with primary closure versus venous patch closure or PTFE patch closure, but there was no statistical difference for RIND, TIA, or perioperative death (Table 12.1).
- Overall rates of early and long-term strokes were statistically higher in patients with primary closure. The cumulative stroke-free survival rate at 48 months was 82% for primary closure, 84% for PTFE patch closure, and 88% for venous patch closure (p < 0.01).
- Primary closure had a significantly higher incidence of recurrent stenosis and occlusion (34%) compared to PTFE (2%) and venous patch

closures (9%). PTFE patch closure had a lower recurrent stenosis rate than venous patch (p < 0.045). Kaplan–Meier analysis showed that freedom from recurrent stenosis at 48 months was 47% for primary closure, 84% for venous patch closure, and 96% for PTFE patch closure (p < 0.001).

Table 12.1 Perioperative mortality/morbidity and long-term recurrent stenosis

	Primary closure (PC) (n = 135)	PTFE closure (PTFE-P) (n = 134)	Vein patch closure (VPC) (n = 130)
Ipsilateral stroke*	6	1	0
Ipsilateral RIND	1	2	1
Ipsilateral TIA	3	3	3
Death	2	0	2
Recurrent stenosis (>50%)[†]	45	3	11

*PC vs. all patching (vein and PTFE), p = 0.007; PC vs. VPC, p = 0.0165; VPC vs. PTFE-P, p = 0.51.
[†]PC vs. patching, p < 0.001; PC vs. PTFE-P, p < 0.001; PC vs. VPC, p < 0.001; PTFE-P vs. VPC, p = 0.045.

Criticisms and Limitations: Advocates of primary closure have argued that patients with large arteries or short arteriotomy can be safely operated on with that technique. However, this subgroup of patients was not analyzed in this study. Another limitation of the trial was that it was a single-center study with a low rate of events.

Other Relevant Studies and Information

- A Cochrane review in 2009 concluded that the current evidence suggests that carotid patching may reduce the risk of perioperative arterial conclusion, ipsilateral stroke, and restenosis.[2]
- Another Cochrane review published in 2021 studied the effects of different patches on perioperative outcomes and concluded that bovine pericardial patch may reduce the risk of perioperative fatal stroke, death, and infection compared to other synthetic patches.[3]
- The European Society for Vascular Surgery guidelines recommend the routine use of patching rather than primary closure.[4]
- The Society for Vascular Surgery clinical practice guidelines also recommend routine carotid patching.[5]

Summary and Implications: This randomized controlled trial showed that, among patients undergoing CEA, patching in general is superior to primary closure in lowering the incidence of perioperative stroke as well as reducing the rate of significant recurrent carotid artery stenosis over the long term.

CLINICAL CASE: PATCH ANGIOPLASTY DURING CEA

Case History

A 75-year-old female patient is due to have a CEA following a recent TIA. During the consenting process, you explain to her that you will repair the artery with a patch angioplasty. She asks what the benefit is of patching the artery.

Suggested Answer

The evidence, as shown by this study, suggests that there is benefit with patching over primary closure as it reduces perioperative strokes in addition to reducing the rate of significant restenosis in the longer term. Therefore, patching offers both early and late benefits compared to primary closure. The randomized controlled trial also showed that women with primary closure had a higher recurrent stenosis rate than men (46% vs. 23%, p = 0.008). She underwent a successful CEA with a vein patch.

References

1. AbuRahma AF, Robinson PA, Saiedy S, et al. Prospective randomized trial of carotid endarterectomy with primary closure and patch angioplasty with saphenous vein, jugular vein, and polytetrafluoroethylene: Long-term follow-up. *J Vasc Surg.* 1998;27(2):222–232.
2. Rerkasem K, Rothwell PM. Patches of different types for carotid patch angioplasty. *Cochrane Database Syst Rev.* 2010;2010(3):CD000071.
3. Orrapin S, Benyakorn T, Howard DP, et al. Patches of different types for carotid patch angioplasty. *Cochrane Database Syst Rev.* 2021;2(2):CD000071.
4. Naylor AR, Ricco JB, de Borst GJ, et al. Management of atherosclerotic carotid and vertebral artery disease: 2017 clinical practice guidelines of the European Society for Vascular Surgery (ESVS). *Eur J Vasc Endovasc Surg.* 2018;55(1):3–81.
5. AbuRahma AF, Avgerinos EM, Chang RW, et al. Society for Vascular Surgery clinical practice guidelines for management of extracranial cerebrovascular diseases. *J Vasc Surg.* 2022;75(1S):26S–98S.

Thoracic Outlet

JULIEN AL SHAKARCHI AND ANDREW GARNHAM

13

A Decade of Excellent Outcomes After Surgical Intervention in 538 Patients with Thoracic Outlet Syndrome

Results of this surgical series of [neurogenic thoracic outlet syndrome], [venous thoracic outlet syndrome], and [arterial thoracic outlet syndrome] are extremely positive due to appropriate selection of patients with [neurogenic thoracic outlet syndrome], use of a standard protocol for patients with [venous thoracic outlet syndrome], and expedient intervention in patients with [arterial thoracic outlet syndrome].

ORLANDO ET AL.

Research Question: What are the outcomes of a large cohort of patients who underwent first rib resection (FRR) for thoracic outlet syndrome (TOS) during a period of 10 years?

Funding: No external funding

Year Study Began: 2003

Year Study Published: 2014

Study Location: Single clinical center from the US

Who Was Studied: All patients with clinical signs and symptoms of neurogenic thoracic outlet syndrome (NTOS) without symptomatic relief after 8 weeks of physical therapy, and patients who presented with vascular TOS subtypes with venous thrombosis, venous compression, arterial occlusion, embolization, or aneurysm

Who Was Excluded: Patients with postoperative follow-up of <1 year

Patients: 538

Study Overview: This was a large cohort study assessing the outcomes of patients undergoing FRR for all subtypes of TOS (venous, arterial, and neurogenic). Diagnosis of NTOS was based on symptomatic presentation, physical examination, and no evidence of a more likely cause.

Study Intervention: Patients with NTOS received Botox or lidocaine blocks of the anterior scalene muscle to confirm that they would benefit from surgical intervention. Duplex ultrasonography was the diagnostic modality of choice to confirm the diagnosis of venous thoracic outlet syndrome (VTOS) and arterial thoracic outlet syndrome (ATOS).

Follow-up: Mean duration of 13.4 months

Endpoints: For patients with NTOS, the central outcome was symptom control. For patients with VTOS and ATOS, positive outcomes were defined as vessel patency of the ipsilateral subclavian vein or artery visualized at last follow-up on duplex scan.

RESULTS

- 538 patients underwent 594 FRR procedures for indications of NTOS (n = 308 [52%]), VTOS (n = 261 [44%]), and ATOS (n = 25 [4%]) (Table 13.1).
- 67% of FRR procedures were performed on female patients, with a mean age of 33 years (range 10–71 years).
- 138 (23%) intraoperative pneumothoraces were treated with placement of intraoperative chest tubes, which were removed the next day. Other complications included eight (1.3%) wound infections, six hematomas, two hemothoraces, and two vein injuries.
- The clinical outcome was positive in 93% of patients treated for NTOS, 97% for VTOS, and 100% for ATOS.

- Over time, there was an increasing trend of surgical treatment for children and adolescents with TOS.

Table 13.1 Clinical outcomes following FRR

Characteristics	Positive outcome n (%)	Total number
All TOS	530 (95%)	557
NTOS	281 (93%)	301
VTOS	225 (97%)	232
ATOS	24 (100%)	24

Criticisms and Limitations: This was a specialized single-center study with an experienced team. The observed results might not be achievable in other settings.

Lidocaine/Botox blocks are not available in every unit; therefore, the diagnosis of NTOS might be more challenging. In addition, these tests might also cause false-negative results if the muscle has become fibrotic secondary to repetitive trauma.

In this study, the researchers did not clearly define what was a positive outcome following FRR for NTOS. There was also no long-term follow-up for this cohort of patients in terms of symptom recurrence.

Other Relevant Studies and Information

- The Society for Vascular Surgery has developed reporting standards for TOS to produce consistency in diagnosis, description of treatment, and assessment of results.[2]
- The European Society for Vascular Surgery guidelines on the management of venous thrombosis recommend that for patients with upper extremity deep vein thrombosis treated by early thrombus removal, FRR may be considered if there is clear evidence of VTOS.[3]
- A study on the surgical management of TOS in adolescents concluded that surgical intervention for TOS in the adolescent population results in excellent outcomes in the short term. However, recurrence of mild symptoms in this population is common and patients need to be counseled clearly about this prior to surgical intervention.[4]

Summary and Implications: Results of this surgical series of patients with NTOS, VTOS, and ATOS showed that with careful patient selection, a standardized protocol for patient with VTOS, expedient intervention in patients with ATOS, and an experienced team, outcomes after a mean duration of 13.4 months are generally favorable.

CLINICAL CASE: NTOS

Case History

A 45-year-old secretary attends your clinic with a complaint of left arm pain, paresthesia down the arm along the ulnar distribution, and weakness of grip, especially on arm elevation. She tells you that she has been suffering from this for many years but no one has been able to diagnose her. How would you manage this patient?

Suggested Answer

I would take a full history from the patient and perform a clinical examination to exclude any other diagnosis. I would perform specific maneuvers, including an elevated arm stress test (also known as the Roos test), upper limb tension test, and Adson's test. I would order a cervical spine x-ray to exclude a cervical rib. Once a clinical diagnosis has been made, I would refer the patient for physiotherapy and reassess for symptomatic relief. If she is still symptomatic after a period of physiotherapy, I would recommend an ultrasound-guided Botox or lidocaine block of the anterior scalene muscle. If she benefits from the block, I would counsel her about the benefits and risks of surgery.

References

1. Orlando MS, Likes KC, Mirza S, et al. A decade of excellent outcomes after surgical intervention in 538 patients with thoracic outlet syndrome. *J Am Coll Surg*. 2015;220(5):934–939.
2. Illig KA, Donahue D, Duncan A, et al. Reporting standards of the Society for Vascular Surgery for thoracic outlet syndrome. *J Vasc Surg*. 2016;64(3):e23–e35.
3. Kakkos SK, Gohel M, Baekgaard N, et al. European Society for Vascular Surgery (ESVS) 2021 clinical practice guidelines on the management of venous thrombosis. *Eur J Vasc Endovasc Surg*. 2021;61(1):9–82.
4. Al Shakarchi J, Jaipersad A, Morgan R, Pherwani A. Early and late outcomes of surgery for neurogenic thoracic outlet syndrome in adolescents. *Ann Vasc Surg*. 2020;63:332–335.

14

A Systematic Review and Meta-Analysis for the Management of Paget–Schroetter Syndrome

Paget–Schroetter syndrome is the most common cause for upper extremity [deep vein thrombosis] and needs to be treated promptly to
avoid potentially long-term debilitating sequelae.

KAROLANIS ET AL.

Research Question: Is anticoagulation or thrombolysis with decompression
safe and efficacious for the treatment of Paget–Schroetter syndrome (PSS)?[1]

Funding: No external funding

Year Range for Searches: 1989–2019

Year Study Published: 2021

Number of Studies Included in Systematic Review: 25 studies

Studies Included: Studies reporting on PSS defined by spontaneous thrombosis or thrombosis after strenuous activities of the axillary/subclavian veins
were considered eligible. Only studies with >10 patients were included in the
meta-analysis.

Studies Excluded: Studies focusing on other reasons for upper extremity deep
vein thrombosis (DVT), studies without a clear indication of PSS, or studies that

did not provide numerical data were excluded from the analysis. Studies that referred to reoperations after PSS were also excluded as well as studies with duplicate data.

Patients: 1,511

Study Overview: A systematic review and a meta-analysis of the management of PSS were carried out to extract information on the epidemiologic, etiologic, and clinical characteristics of PSS, along with radiologic findings and treatment outcomes. A subgroup meta-analysis was also performed to investigate studies for patients who had initial thrombolysis. They were then divided into three groups: studies reporting data for patients who had additional first rib resection (FRR), studies reporting data for patients who had additional FRR and endogenous balloon venoplasty (FRR + venoplasty), and studies reporting data for patients who did not have any further intervention (no FRR).

Follow-up: Mean follow-up 42 months

Endpoints: Outcome measures included:
- Rates of complete, partial, and no thrombus resolution after thrombolysis and after anticoagulation
- Complications, including bleeding, pneumothorax, and nerve injury
- Complete, partial, and no thrombus resolution during follow-up; the investigators also estimated rates of asymptomatic patients, along with patients who sustained rethrombosis during the follow-up period

RESULTS

- Of the 1,511 patients included in the systematic review, 1,177 (77.9%) had thrombolysis, 658 (43.5%) had anticoagulation, and 1293 (85.6%) had decompression therapy of the thoracic outlet. The median time between diagnosis and thrombolysis was 5.6 days.
- Complete thrombus resolution was estimated at about 78.1% (95% confidence interval [CI], 66.04–88.39; 15 studies) of the patients after thrombolysis. After anticoagulation, a total of 40.7% of the patients (95% CI, 11.06–73.57; six studies) had complete thrombus resolution.
- Regarding the subgroup meta-analysis, in the FRR group, the vein patency and symptom relief outcomes at last follow-up were 97.9% (95% CI, 90.55–100) and 98.0% (95% CI, 94.33–99.96), respectively. In the

FRR + venoplasty group, the vein patency was 93.3% (95% CI, 80.15–99.99) and symptom relief was 99.5% (95% CI, 93.26–100). For patients who did not have FRR after clot lysis, the vein patency was 63.6% (95% CI, 20.17–97.40) and the symptom relief rate was 70.7% (95% CI, 40.35–94.03).

- Complications following FRR were not uncommon and were estimated at 4.9% (95% CI, 2.15–8.38) for postoperative bleeding, 6.0% (95% CI, 1.76–12.01) for pneumothorax, and 3.7% (95% CI, 0.10–10.25) for nerve injury.

Criticisms and Limitations: All studies were retrospective, and only six studies contained a significant number of participants (>50). This is likely to lead to publication bias as it is less likely that a study with unfavorable outcomes would get published. Therefore, real-world practice might have different results, with less symptomatic relief and more complications.

Other Relevant Studies and Information

- A recent case series documenting the novel use of robot-assisted transthoracic FRR with only three trocars has shown the technique to be a feasible minimally invasive approach for FRR in the management of venous thoracic outlet syndrome. This technique enables the surgeon to perform venolysis under direct 3D vision with good patency and long-term functional outcome.[2]
- The European Society for Vascular Surgery guidelines on the management of venous thrombosis recommend that in selected young and active patients with upper extremity DVT with severe symptoms, thrombolysis may be considered within the first 2 weeks. The guidelines also recommend that for patients with upper extremity DVT treated by early thrombus removal, FRR may be considered if there is clear evidence of venous thoracic outlet syndrome.[3]

Summary and Implications: Although no randomized controlled data were available, this analysis among patients with PSS strongly suggests higher rates of thrombus and symptom resolution with thrombolysis, followed by FRR. A prospective randomized trial is really needed to compare anticoagulation with thrombolysis and to assess when and if decompression of the thoracic outlet is required.

CLINICAL CASE: UPPER LIMB DVT
FOLLOWING EXERCISE

Case History

A 25-year-old gym enthusiast presents to the emergency department with a very swollen left arm. He has an elevated D-dimer level and an ultrasound duplex reveals an extensive thrombus in his axillary vein. How would you manage this patient?

Suggested Answer

This patient should be started on anticoagulation, compression, and arm elevation. Catheter-directed thrombolysis should be considered early (within 2 weeks of the event) if no improvement is seen with conservative management as the patient is young and very symptomatic. Following successful thrombolysis, an FRR is performed during the same admission, and at the time of surgery the patency of the vein is checked. The patient makes a good postoperative recovery and a follow-up venogram showed a fully patent vein.

References

1. Karaolanis G, Antonopoulos CN, Koutsias SG, et al. A systematic review and meta-analysis for the management of Paget–Schroetter syndrome. *J Vasc Surg Venous Lymphat Disord.* 2021;9(3):801–810.
2. Hoexum F, Jongkind V, Coveliers HM, et al. Robot-assisted transthoracic first rib resection for venous thoracic outlet syndrome. *Vascular.* 2022;30(2):217–224.
3. Kakkos SK, Gohel M, Baekgaard N, et al. European Society for Vascular Surgery (ESVS) 2021 clinical practice guidelines on the management of venous thrombosis. *Eur J Vasc Endovasc Surg.* 2021;61(1):9–82.

Thoracic Aortic Disease

JULIEN AL SHAKARCHI AND DONALD ADAM

15

Randomized Comparison of Strategies for Type B Aortic Dissection

The Investigation of Stent Grafts in Aortic Dissection (INSTEAD) Trial

[Thoracic endovascular aneurysm repair] failed to improve 2-year survival and adverse event rates despite favorable aortic remodeling.
THE INSTEAD INVESTIGATORS

Research Question: Is there any benefit in endovascular stent grafting as an adjunct to best medical therapy (BMT) in patients with uncomplicated type B aortic dissection?[1]

Funding: Medtronic Bakken Research Institute and the Institutional Research Unit at Rostock University

Year Study Began: 2003

Year Study Published: 2009

Study Location: Seven clinical centers from Germany, Italy, and France

Who Was Studied: Inclusion criteria were adult patients with uncomplicated type B aortic dissection.

Who Was Excluded: Exclusion criteria included presence of indications for endovascular or open surgery (such as a descending thoracic aorta of diameter 6 cm), recurrence of acute complications, or anatomic contraindication to thoracic endovascular aneurysm repair (TEVAR).

Patients: 140

Study Overview

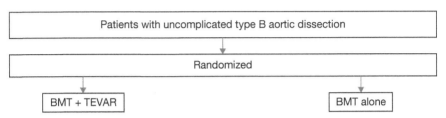

Figure 15.1 Design of INSTEAD randomized controlled trial

Study Intervention: Patients were randomly assigned to TEVAR + BMT or to BMT alone.

Follow-up: 2 years

Endpoints: *Primary outcome measure:* All-cause death at 2 years. *Secondary outcome measures:* Aorta-related death, a composite endpoint of progressive aortic pathology (including crossover/conversion or additional endovascular or open surgery for rupture, expansion, or malperfusion), and morphological evidence of aortic remodeling.

RESULTS

- The mean age of patients was 60 years old and 84% were male. The time interval between onset of dissection and randomization was similar between groups, with a median of 45 (BMT) and 39 days (TEVAR + BMT). The median interval between randomization and stent-graft placement was 12 days.
- There was no difference in all-cause mortality, with a 2-year cumulative survival rate of 95.6% with BMT versus 88.9% with TEVAR + BMT (p = 0.15).
- There was no significant difference in aorta-related death rate (p = 0.44) or the risk for the combined endpoint of aorta-related death (rupture)

and progression (including conversion or additional endovascular or open surgery) (p = 0.65) (Table 15.1).

- Three neurological adverse events occurred in the TEVAR + BMT group (one paraplegia, one stroke, and one transient paraparesis) versus one case of paraparesis with BMT alone.
- Aortic remodeling (with true-lumen recovery and thoracic false-lumen thrombosis) occurred in 91.3% of patients with TEVAR versus 19.4% of those who received BMT alone (p = 0.001).

Table 15.1 Events in BMT and BMT + TEVAR groups

	BMT	BMT + TEVAR
Overall death n (%)	3 (4.4)	8 (11.1)
Aorta-related deaths n (%)	2 (2.9)	4 (5.6)
Secondary interventions n (%)	15 (22.1)	13 (18.1)
Persistent paraplegia/paraparesis n (%)	1 (1.4)	2 (2.8)
Major stroke n (%)	0 (0)	2 (2.8)

Criticisms and Limitations

- Potential benefits of TEVAR may emerge in some patients beyond the 2-year window of the INSTEAD trial.
- The trial included patients with chronic dissection ranging from 2 to 52 weeks after onset. Some clinicians consider that patients benefit more from TEVAR during the sub-acute phase (2–12 weeks) rather than at a later stage.
- TEVAR technology and operator skills have evolved since the trial, which is likely to have led to a reduction in procedure-related adverse events.

Other Relevant Studies and Information

- The INSTEAD-XL study showed that TEVAR + BMT is associated with improved 5-year aorta-specific survival and delayed disease progression.[2]
- The 2014 European Society for Cardiology guidelines on the diagnosis and treatment of aortic diseases state that in uncomplicated type B aortic dissection, TEVAR should be considered.[3]
- The 2017 European Society for Vascular Surgery guidelines on the management of descending thoracic aorta diseases state that in patients who are at risk of further aortic complications and who have suitable

anatomy for TEVAR, endovascular repair of uncomplicated type B aortic dissections should be considered in the sub-acute phase if performed in dedicated centers.[4]

Summary and Implications: In this randomized study on elective stent-graft placement in survivors of uncomplicated type B aortic dissection, TEVAR failed to improve 2-year survival and adverse event rates versus standard medical therapy despite being associated with favorable aortic remodeling.

CLINICAL CASE: UNCOMPLICATED TYPE B AORTIC DISSECTION

Case History

A 69-year-old man is admitted to the hospital with acute chest pain radiating to his back. A computed tomographic (CT) angiogram confirms a type B aortic dissection with no adverse features. He is treated medically and is discharged at day 5 with oral antihypertensive medications. He comes back to your clinic following a 6-week CT angiogram of his aorta showing no changes in his morphology. How would you manage this patient?

Suggested Answer

The patient should continue with BMT. He should be counseled about the management options with either medical treatment alone with regular imaging or thoracic stenting with medical treatment. You explain to him that the INSTEAD trial did not show any improvement in survival or adverse events at 2 years; however, there might be some long-term improvement in outcomes. After understanding the possible risks of the procedure (paraplegia, stroke, or death), he decides to continue with medical management and follow-up imaging. At year 5, his thoracic aorta has enlarged to 61 mm on a follow-up CT angiogram and he undergoes a TEVAR without any complications.

References

1. Nienaber CA, Rousseau H, Eggebrecht H, et al. Randomized comparison of strategies for type B aortic dissection: The INvestigation of STEnt Grafts in Aortic Dissection (INSTEAD) trial. *Circulation.* 2009;120(25):2519–2528.
2. Nienaber CA, Kische S, Rousseau H, et al. Endovascular repair of type B aortic dissection: Long-term results of the randomized investigation of stent grafts in aortic dissection trial. *Circ Cardiovasc Interv.* 2013;6(4):407–416.

3. Erbel R, Aboyans V, Boileau C, et al. 2014 ESC guidelines on the diagnosis and treatment of aortic diseases: Document covering acute and chronic aortic diseases of the thoracic and abdominal aorta of the adult. The Task Force for the Diagnosis and Treatment of Aortic Diseases of the European Society of Cardiology (ESC). *Eur Heart J.* 2014;35(41):2873–2926.

4. Riambau V, Böckler D, Brunkwall J, et al. Management of descending thoracic aorta diseases: Clinical practice guidelines of the European Society for Vascular Surgery (ESVS). *Eur J Vasc Endovasc Surg.* 2017;53(1):4–52.

16

Outcomes of 3,309 Thoracoabdominal Aortic Aneurysm Repairs

Data suggest that open [thoracoabdominal aortic aneurysm] repair performed at an experienced center can produce respectable outcomes.

COSELLI ET AL.

Research Question: What are the long-term outcomes of open surgical repair of thoracoabdominal aortic aneurysms (TAAAs)?[1]

Funding: None

Years Patients Were Treated: 1986–2014

Year Study Published: 2016

Study Location: Single clinical center from the US

Who Was Studied: Adult patients with an extent I–IV TAAA were included.

Who Was Excluded: Patients who were unable or unavailable to provide consent for the protocol were excluded from the study.

Patients: 3,309

Study Overview: This was a descriptive retrospective data analysis to identify all adult patients who had undergone extent I–IV open TAAA repair between

1986 and 2006 and of a prospective database from 2006 to 2014 and describe the outcomes.

Study Intervention: Repairs included 914 Crawford extent I, 1,066 extent II, 660 extent III, and 669 extent IV TAAA repairs. The treating surgeons routinely used moderate systemic heparinization (1.0 mg/kg) and mild permissive hypothermia (32°–34°C, nasopharyngeal), and when possible segmental intercostal and lumbar arteries were reattached to the graft. The renal arteries were intermittently perfused with cold (4°C) crystalloid. Operative adjuncts that are generally reserved for more extensive TAAA repairs (i.e., Crawford extents I and II) included cerebrospinal fluid drainage and selective perfusion of the celiac and superior mesenteric arteries.

Endpoints: The outcomes were operative death, 30-day mortality, paraplegia/paraparesis, renal failure requiring hemodialysis, pulmonary complications, cardiac events, and return to the operating room for control of bleeding.

RESULTS

- Of 3,309 repairs, 2043 (61.7%) were performed in men with a mean patient age of 67 years. Cardiovascular risk factors included hypertension (84.8%), chronic lung disease (39.2%), coronary artery disease (37.2%), peripheral vascular disease (25.8%), cerebrovascular disease (17.4%), and diabetes (7.9%).
- The operative mortality rate was 6.2% in elective repairs (n = 2,586) and 12.2% in urgent or emergency repairs (n = 723). The operative mortality was higher after extent II and III repairs (9.5% and 8.8%, respectively) than in extents I and IV (5.9% and 5.4%, respectively) (Table 16.1).
- Pulmonary complications occurred in 35.8%, with cardiac events in 26%, renal failure requiring hemodialysis in 7.6%, permanent spinal cord injury in 5.4%, stroke in 3%, and reoperation for control of bleeding in 3.3%.
- Estimated survival was 83.5% at 1 year, 63.6% at 5 years, 36.8% at 10 years, and 18.3% at 15 years.

Table 16.1 POSTOPERATIVE MORBIDITY AND MORTALITY

Event	All (n = 3,309)	Extent I (n = 914)	Extent II (n = 1,066)	Extent III (n = 660)	Extent IV (n = 669)
Operative death	249 (7.5%)	54 (5.9%)	101 (9.5%)	58 (8.8%)	36 (5.4%)
Cerebral complication	267 (8.1%)	74 (8.1%)	124 (11.6%)	40 (6.1%)	29 (4.3%)
Permanent spinal cord deficit	178 (5.4%)	31 (3.4%)	85 (8.0%)	46 (7.0%)	16 (2.4%)
Renal failure requiring permanent dialysis	189 (5.7%)	29 (3.2%)	78 (7.3%)	43 (6.5%)	39 (5.8%)
Cardiac complication	860 (26.0%)	221 (24.2%)	334 (31.3%)	158 (23.9%)	147 (22.0%)
Respiratory complication	1185 (35.8%)	347 (38.0%)	455 (42.7%)	223 (33.8%)	160 (23.9%)

Criticisms and Limitations: As with all retrospective studies, the analysis cannot consider any confounding variables. It is also likely that the retrospective data pre-2006 did not fully capture all preoperative characteristics or postoperative complications.

This is a single-center study from a large experienced US aortic center and may not be representative of outcomes in other settings or among other populations.

Other Relevant Studies and Information

- A single-center study from an experienced UK center reported excellent outcomes with low perioperative morbidity and mortality and good medium-term outcomes for elective fenestrated and branched endovascular repair of TAAAs.[2]
- A recently published systematic review investigating the outcomes of endovascular and open TAAA showed that perioperative mortality rates were similar; however, the endovascular cohort had more comorbidities.[3]
- The 2017 European Society for Vascular Surgery guidelines state that open or endovascular repair should be considered for patients at low to moderate surgical risk, with an atherosclerotic or degenerative TAAA

60 mm or larger in diameter, rapid aneurysm enlargement (>10 mm/ year), or aneurysm-related symptoms.[4]

Summary and Implications: The results from the study suggest that open TAAA repair, when performed at a large-volume, experienced center, can produce respectable outcomes.

CLINICAL CASE: EXTENT III TAAA

Case History
A 55-year-old man is referred to your clinic with an incidental finding of a TAAA following an ultrasound. He has undergone a computed tomographic angiogram, which confirms an extent III TAAA. His past medical history consists of well-controlled hypertension. He is active and plays tennis every weekend. How would you manage this patient?

Suggested Answer
This patient should be referred to a large tertiary unit with expertise in both open and endovascular TAAA repair. He needs to have an anesthetic assessment with cardiac and respiratory testing. Following a multidisciplinary team meeting, he is counseled for both procedures as he is found to have good physiological reserve. He opts for an open repair, and although he develops a postoperative chest infection, he makes a good recovery and is discharged home on day 10.

References

1. Coselli JS, LeMaire SA, Preventza O, et al. Outcomes of 3309 thoracoabdominal aortic aneurysm repairs. *J Thorac Cardiovasc Surg.* 2016;151(5):1323–1337.
2. Juszczak MT, Murray A, Koutsoumpelis A, et al. Elective fenestrated and branched endovascular thoraco-abdominal aortic repair with supracoeliac sealing zones and without prophylactic cerebrospinal fluid drainage: Early and medium-term outcomes. *Eur J Vasc Endovasc Surg.* 2019;57(5):639–648.
3. Rocha RV, Lindsay TF, Friedrich JO, et al. Systematic review of contemporary outcomes of endovascular and open thoracoabdominal aortic aneurysm repair. *J Vasc Surg.* 2020;71(4):1396–1412.
4. Riambau V, Böckler D, Brunkwall J, et al. Management of descending thoracic aorta diseases: Clinical practice guidelines of the European Society for Vascular Surgery (ESVS). *Eur J Vasc Endovasc Surg.* 2017;53(1):4–52.

17

Long-Term Results of Endovascular Repair for Descending Thoracic Aortic Aneurysms

This study suggests that thoracic endovascular aortic repair for degenerative descending thoracic aortic aneurysms is safe, effective, and durable at 12 years of follow-up.

RANNEY ET AL.

Research Question: What are the long-term outcomes of thoracic endovascular aortic repair (TEVAR) for descending thoracic aortic aneurysms (DTaas)?[1]

Funding: None

Years Patients Were Treated: 2005–2016

Year Study Published: 2018

Study Location: Single clinical center from the US

Who Was Studied: The study included adult patients who underwent TEVAR within instruction for use for the indication of DTAA.

Who Was Excluded: Patients were excluded if they were undergoing hybrid procedures including arch or visceral debranching, TEVAR for dissection or intramural hematoma, and any endograft landing in Dacron replaced aorta.

Patients: 192

Study Overview: A retrospective observational analysis was performed using a prospectively maintained database from a single referral aortic center to identify all adult patients undergoing TEVAR for DTAA between March 2005 and April 2016.

Study Intervention: Preoperative TEVAR planning was performed using the TeraRecon system with centerline measurements of flow lumen diameter by computed tomographic (CT) angiography to assess landing zones as well as iliofemoral access vessels. All CTAs included the base of the neck to allow assessment of the common carotid and vertebral arteries. Routine postoperative surveillance consisted of CT angiography at 1, 6, and 12 months after TEVAR and annually thereafter. In addition, 3-month follow-up assessments and imaging were obtained in patients with an endoleak identified at 1 month, if the decision for initial endoleak observation was made.

Follow-up: Mean duration of 69 months

Endpoints: Short-term outcomes were 30-day and in-hospital mortality, stroke, new permanent dialysis, and permanent paraparesis and paraplegia. Long-term outcomes were survival and rate of reintervention secondary to endoleak.

RESULTS

- The mean age was 71.1 years; 55.7% of patients were male. All aneurysms were attributed to degenerative atherosclerotic disease without suspicion of connective tissue disorder. The mean aortic diameter was 5.9 cm.
- 75% of cases were performed electively. Of the 25% of cases (n = 48) performed urgently or emergently, 10 presented with rupture and the remainder were symptomatic. Partial or complete left subclavian artery coverage occurred in 88 patients (45.8%), of whom 12 (13.6%) underwent concomitant revascularization via left carotid–subclavian artery bypass (Table 17.1).

Table 17.1 OPERATIVE CHARACTERISTICS

Operative variable	
Elective n (%)	144 (75%)
Fusiform n (%)	106 (55.2%)
Left subclavian artery coverage n (%)	88 (45.8%)
Maximum aortic diameter cm	5.9
Endograft used n	2
Prophylactic cerebrospinal fluid drain n (%)	24 (12.5%)

- Rates of 30-day and in-hospital mortality, stroke, permanent dialysis, and permanent paraparesis or paraplegia were 4.7%, 2.1%, 0.5%, and 0.5% respectively. Notably, the 30-day and in-hospital survival rate was 90% among the 10 patients presenting with aortic rupture.
- Overall and aorta-specific survival rates at 141 months (11.8 years) were 45.7% and 96.2%, respectively. During long-term follow-up, endovascular reintervention was required in 14 patients (7.3%) owing to type I (n = 10), type II (n = 2), and type III (n = 2) endoleak.

Criticisms and Limitations: This is a retrospective observational study, which means the analysis might have missed confounding variables. Also, the results presented in this study represent outcomes from a high-volume referral center and may not be generalizable to other centers. Clinical practice would also have changed over the long study period, and this may have had an impact on the outcomes.

Other Relevant Studies and Information

- The 2014 European Society for Cardiology guidelines on the diagnosis and treatment of aortic diseases state that TEVAR should be considered in patients who have a DTAA with a maximal diameter of ≥55 mm rather than surgery.[2]
- The 2021 Society for Vascular Surgery recommends TEVAR as the preferred approach to treat elective DTAA, given its reduced morbidity and length of stay as well as short-term mortality.[3]
- The 2017 European Society for Vascular Surgery guidelines state that in patients with favorable anatomy, TEVAR should be considered for DTAA >60 mm in diameter.[4]

Summary and Implications: Long-term aorta-specific survival after on-label endovascular repair of degenerative descending thoracic aneurysms is excellent, with sustained protection from rupture and a low rate of reintervention for endoleak. Endovascular repair should be considered the treatment of choice for this pathology.

CLINICAL CASE: DTAA

Case History
A 70-year-old man is referred to the vascular clinic with an incidental finding of DTAA following a CT scan obtained during an in-hospital admission with

pneumonia. He has made a full recovery from the pneumonia and he is generally medically well with good mobility. How would you manage this patient?

Suggested Answer

This patient needs to have formal CT angiography of his whole aorta. Using computer software reconstruction, the aneurysm measures 60 mm in diameter and you decide that the left subclavian artery will require coverage for your proximal landing seal zone. Therefore, you counsel the patient about having a left carotid–subclavian bypass with a TEVAR and explain to him that TEVAR has been shown to have an excellent long-term outcome for his pathology. He agrees to have a procedure and is discharged home 3 days after surgery, having made a full recovery.

References

1. Ranney DN, Cox ML, Yerokun BA, et al. Long-term results of endovascular repair for descending thoracic aortic aneurysms. *J Vasc Surg*. 2018;67(2):363–368.
2. Erbel R, Aboyans V, Boileau C, et al. 2014 ESC guidelines on the diagnosis and treatment of aortic diseases: Document covering acute and chronic aortic diseases of the thoracic and abdominal aorta of the adult. The Task Force for the Diagnosis and Treatment of Aortic Diseases of the European Society of Cardiology (ESC). *Eur Heart J*. 2014;35(41):2873–2926.
3. Upchurch GR Jr, Escobar GA, Azizzadeh A, et al. Society for Vascular Surgery clinical practice guidelines of thoracic endovascular aortic repair for descending thoracic aortic aneurysms. *J Vasc Surg*. 2021;73(1S):55S–83S.
4. Riambau V, Böckler D, Brunkwall J, et al. Management of descending thoracic aorta diseases: Clinical practice guidelines of the European Society for Vascular Surgery (ESVS). *Eur J Vasc Endovasc Surg*. 2017;53(1):4–52.

SECTION 5

Abdominal Aortic Disease

JULIEN AL SHAKARCHI

18

Multicenter Aneurysm Screening Study (MASS)

Cost-Effectiveness Analysis of Screening for Abdominal Aortic Aneurysms Based on 4-Year Results from a Randomized Controlled Trial

The projected cost per life-year gained after 10 years was £8,000, which is substantially lower than the perceived [National Health Service] threshold value.

THE MASS INVESTIGATORS

Research Question: Does ultrasound screening for abdominal aortic aneurysm (AAA) decrease mortality, and is it cost-effective?[1]

Funding: UK Medical Research Council and the Department of Health

Year Study Began: 1997

Year Study Published: 2002

Study Location: Four clinical centers from the UK

Who Was Studied: Men aged 65–74 years identified from Health Authority and family doctor patient lists were included in this study.

Who Was Excluded: Patients identified by their family doctor as being terminally ill, having serious comorbidities, or having undergone a previous AAA repair were excluded.

Patients: 67,800

Study Overview

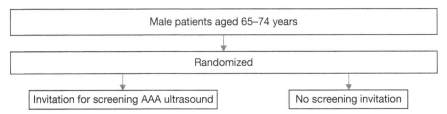

Figure 18.1 Design of MASS randomized controlled trial

Study Intervention: Patients were randomly assigned to either receive an invitation for a screening abdominal ultrasound (invited group) or not (control group). Men with normal aortas (<3 cm in diameter) were not rescanned. Patients with aortas measuring 3.0–4.4 cm were rescanned annually, while patients with aortas measuring 4.5–5.4 cm were rescanned at 3-month intervals. Urgent referral to surgery was recommended for patients with aortas measuring ≥5.5 cm and those with growth of ≥1 cm per year.

Follow-up: Mean of 4.1 years follow-up for men with AAA ≥3 cm

Endpoints: The main outcome measure was cost-effectiveness as the incremental cost per additional life-year gained.

RESULTS

- 80% (27,147/33,839) of men invited accepted the invitation to screen, with 1,333 (4.9% of those scanned) having AAAs detected. The initial screening generated 4,735 follow-up or recall scans. The mean cost of screening per patient randomized in the intervention group was £23.23.
- While those in the invited group had fewer emergency operations than those in the control group (23 vs. 53), the former had a higher rate of elective surgery (307 vs. 85).
- The mean cost including any related readmissions within 12 months for elective aneurysm repair was £6,909 compared with £11,176 for

emergency surgery. The mean cost per patient of surgery was £76.64 in the intervention group and £35.93 in the control group.

- The screening group had 58 aneurysm-related deaths and the control group had 105 aneurysm-related deaths up to 4 years. The mean survival time free from mortality related to AAA was thus greater in the intervention group than the control group, the mean difference being 0.82 days per patient over 4 years (0.16 to 1.47 days).

- This gives an estimated incremental cost-effectiveness ratio at 4 years of £28,400 per life-year gained. The cost-effectiveness ratio at 10 years is estimated to be around £8,000 per life-year saved.

Criticisms and Limitations: The portable ultrasound machine used in this study represents outdated technology; therefore, more accurate measurements can now be made and the results might be different now.

A small proportion of patients' aortas (about 1%) were not visualized on ultrasound, and these patients were not rescreened. Some aneurysms could have been missed due to this.

Other Relevant Studies and Information

- The VIVA study, which randomized 50,156 men aged 65–74 to screening for AAA or peripheral arterial disease, showed a reduction in all-cause mortality.[2]
- The Society for Vascular Surgery (SVS) recommends a one-time ultrasound screening for men and women aged 65–75 years with a history of tobacco use.[3]
- The European Society for Vascular Surgery (ESVS) 2019 clinical practice guidelines on the management of abdominal aorto-iliac artery aneurysms recommend screening for men over the age of 65 years.[4]

Summary and Implications: AAA screening can decrease aneurysm-related mortality rates. Even at 4 years the cost-effectiveness of AAA screening was shown to have reached acceptability according to current National Health Service thresholds, and this is likely to increase further at 10 years. Since this landmark study, screening for AAA has been implemented in many countries, including the UK.

CLINICAL CASE: SCREENING FOR AAA

Case History

A 69-year-old male presents to your clinic asking about screening for AAA. He is an ex-smoker with a history of hypertension. He is independent and medically well. His older brother has recently passed away from a ruptured AAA at the age of 73 years. How would you advise this patient?

Suggested Answer

The MASS trial has shown that screening in all men aged 65–74 decreases aneurysm-related mortality and is cost-effective. He has two risk factors for AAA, with a family history of AAA rupture and a history of tobacco use. You would advise him that he would benefit from screening and an ultrasound of his aorta should be requested as per SVS and ESVS guidelines.

References

1. Multicentre Aneurysm Screening Study Group. Multicentre Aneurysm Screening Study (MASS): Cost-effectiveness analysis of screening for abdominal aortic aneurysms based on four-year results from randomised controlled trial. *BMJ*. 2002;325(7373):1135.
2. Lindholt JS, Søgaard R. Population screening and intervention for vascular disease in Danish men (VIVA): A randomised controlled trial. *Lancet*. 2017;390(10109):2256–2265.
3. Chaikof EL, Dalman RL, Eskandari MK, et al. The Society for Vascular Surgery practice guidelines on the care of patients with an abdominal aortic aneurysm. *J Vasc Surg*. 2018;67(1):2–77.
4. Wanhainen A, Verzini F, Van Herzeele I, et al. European Society for Vascular Surgery (ESVS) 2019 clinical practice guidelines on the management of abdominal aorto-iliac artery aneurysms. *Eur J Vasc Endovasc Surg*. 2019;57(1):8–93.

19

Long-Term Outcomes of Immediate Repair Compared with Surveillance of Small Abdominal Aortic Aneurysms

United Kingdom Small Aneurysm Trial (UKSAT)

> Ultrasonographic surveillance for small abdominal aortic aneurysms is safe, and early surgery does not provide a long-term survival advantage.
>
> THE UKSAT INVESTIGATORS

Research Question: Does early repair of small abdominal aortic aneurysms (AAAs) improve long-term outcomes?[1]

Funding: Medical Research Council and British Heart Foundation

Year Study Began: 1991

Year Study Published: 2002

Study Location: 93 clinical centers from the UK

Who Was Studied: Patients aged 60–76 with an infrarenal asymptomatic AAA of 4–5.5 cm in diameter were eligible for inclusion.

Who Was Excluded: Patients were excluded if they did not want treatment, were unfit for surgery, were unable to give consent, refused to be randomized, or were unable to attend regular follow-ups.

Patients: 1,090

Study Overview

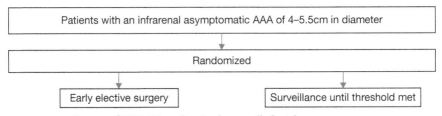

Figure 19.1 Design of UKSAT randomized controlled trial

Study Intervention: Patients were randomly assigned to early elective surgery or ultrasound surveillance. Elective repairs were carried out within 3 months. Ultrasound surveillance was carried out at 6-month intervals until the AAA reached 5–5.5 cm, at which point the interval was shortened to 3 months.

Follow-up: Mean duration of 8 years

Endpoints: Primary outcome measure was mortality. Secondary outcome measures were causes of death and smoking cessation.

RESULTS

- By the end of the trial, 92% of the patients in the early surgery group and 62% of those in the surveillance group had undergone surgical repair of an AAA.
- Survival was initially worse in the early surgery group and was subsequently worse in the surveillance group; the survival curves crossed at about 3 years.
- The mean duration of survival was 6.5 years among patients in the surveillance group and 6.7 years among patients in the early surgery group (p = 0.29).
- The risk of AAA rupture was four times as high in women versus men (hazard ratio, 4.0; 95% percent confidence interval, 2.0–7.9; p < 0.001).
- The rate of smoking cessation was higher in the early surgical group compared to the surveillance group.

Criticisms and Limitations: The trial population mainly consisted of male white patients and therefore the findings might not be generalized to female patients or other ethnic populations.

The elective operative mortality rate of 5.4% in this trial was disappointing and higher than the 2% mortality rate projected in the initial study design.

There might be a subgroup of patients with small AAAs who have a better long-term survival and are more likely to benefit from surgery than a non-selected group of patients.

Other Relevant Studies and Information

- In the Aneurysm Detection and Management (ADAM) study, a similar trial carried out in the US, 1,136 patients were randomized to early elective surgery or surveillance. It found that survival is not improved by elective repair of AAAs <5.5 cm.[2]
- A recently published Cochrane review concluded that there is no advantage to immediate repair for small AAAs regardless of whether open or endovascular repair was used.[3]
- The European Society for Vascular Surgery clinical practice guidelines on the management of abdominal aorto-iliac artery aneurysms recommend repair of a fusiform aneurysm at a size of >5.5 cm.[4]

Summary and Implications: Patients with a small AAA (<5.5 cm) can be monitored with regular ultrasound surveillance as the UKSAT trial showed no survival benefit with early surgery. Female patients were found to have a higher risk of rupture and might benefit from earlier repair, but the threshold has not yet been established.

CLINICAL CASE: MANAGEMENT OF SMALL AAA

Case History

A 69-year-old male patient is being investigated by his urologist for renal stones when an incidental finding of a 4-cm AAA is discovered on a computed tomography scan. He is in excellent health and stopped smoking 10 years ago. He presents to your clinic for your opinion on the management of his AAA. Based on the current evidence, should the patient undergo surgical repair of his aneurysm?

Suggested Answer

The UKSAT showed no long-term survival benefit from early surgical inter-vention, and this finding was confirmed in further randomized controlled trials. He should be entered into a surveillance program until his AAA reaches 5.5 cm unless his aneurysm expands rapidly (1 cm in 1 year) or becomes symptomatic.

References

1. United Kingdom Small Aneurysm Trial Participants. Long-term outcomes of imme-diate repair compared with surveillance of small abdominal aortic aneurysm. *N Engl J Med.* 2002;346(19):1445–1452.
2. Lederle FA, Wilson SE, Johnson GR, et al. Immediate repair compared with surveil-lance of small abdominal aortic aneurysms. *N Engl J Med.* 2002;346(19):1437–1444.
3. Ulug P, Powell JT, Martinez MA, et al. Surgery for small asymptomatic abdominal aortic aneurysms. *Cochrane Database Syst Rev.* 2020;7(7):CD001835.
4. Wanhainen A, Verzini F, Van Herzeele I, et al. European Society for Vascular Surgery (ESVS) 2019 clinical practice guidelines on the management of abdominal aorto-iliac artery aneurysms. *Eur J Vasc Endovasc Surg.* 2019;57(1):8–93.

20

Endovascular Repair Compared with Surveillance for Patients with Small Abdominal Aortic Aneurysms

Positive Impact of Endovascular Options for Treating Aneurysms Early (PIVOTAL) Trial

> Early treatment with endovascular repair and rigorous surveillance with selective aneurysm treatment as indicated both appear to be safe.
>
> THE PIVOTAL INVESTIGATORS

Research Question: Is there an advantage to endovascular repair (EVAR) of small abdominal aortic aneurysms (AAAs) versus surveillance?[1]

Funding: Medtronic Vascular

Year Study Began: 2005

Year Study Published: 2010

Study Location: 65 clinical centers from the US

Who Was Studied: Patients aged 40–90 years with an AAA measuring 4–5 cm in diameter were included if their anatomy was suitable for EVAR and if they were considered to be candidates at low to moderate risk per the Society for Vascular

Surgery (SVS) comorbidity scoring system. To be eligible, patients were also required to have a life expectancy of ≥3 years.

Who Was Excluded: Patients were excluded if the aneurysm anatomy was not amenable to treatment with an endograft or if their comorbidities led to an excessive operative risk. Patients were also excluded if they had any planned surgical or interventional procedure within 30 days after enrollment, a myocardial infarction without revascularization ≤6 months or with revascularization <30 days before enrollment, a known iliac aneurysm ≥3.0 cm, or a known thoracic aneurysm ≥5.0 cm.

Patients: 728

Study Overview

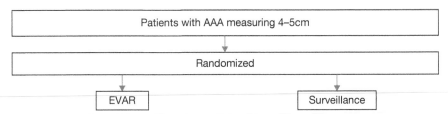

Figure 20.1 Design of PIVOTAL randomized controlled trial

Study Intervention: Patients were randomly assigned to surveillance or EVAR of their AAA. Patients assigned to early EVAR underwent aneurysm repair ≤30 days after randomization using any approved Medtronic endograft system. Individuals in the surveillance group were scheduled to undergo imaging assessments every 6 months.

Follow-up: Mean follow-up was 20 months.

Endpoints: The primary endpoint was the composite of rupture or aneurysm-related death. Secondary outcome measure was aneurysm growth.

RESULTS

- Of the 631 men (86.7%) and 97 women (13.3%), 366 were assigned to early EVAR and 362 to ultrasound surveillance. The mean initial AAA diameter was 4.5 ± 0.3 cm in both groups.

- 322 patients assigned to the early EVAR treatment arm underwent aneurysm repair after a mean of 29.5 days following entry into the study. In the surveillance arm, 112 patients (30.9%) underwent aneurysm repair during follow-up. In the surveillance group the average time from randomization to repair was 370 days, and the average size of the aneurysm at the last imaging report before repair was 4.9 cm (range 4.0–6.5 cm).
- The 30-day operative mortality rate in the early EVAR group was 0.6%. Among the patients in the surveillance group who eventually underwent aneurysm repair, the 30-day operative mortality was 0.9%. At the end of follow-up, mortality was not significantly different (p = 0.98).
- Aneurysm rupture or aneurysm-related death occurred in two patients (0.6%) in the early EVAR group and in two patients (0.6%) in the surveillance group (p = 0.99). Time to rupture or aneurysm-related death was also similar in the two treatment groups.
- Aneurysm growth at 1 year occurred in 35 patients (14.2%) in the surveillance group and in 15 patients (5.7%) in the EVAR group.

Criticisms and Limitations: One of the limitations of the study is that it stopped enrollment early before its planned recruitment of 1,050 patients. The decision was made based on interim analysis showing futility in continuing recruitment to target.

Other Relevant Studies and Information

- The Aneurysm Detection and Management (ADAM) study and the United Kingdom Small Aneurysm Trial (UKSAT; see Chapter 19) were earlier studies comparing open elective surgery to surveillance. They found that survival was not improved by elective repair of AAAs <5.5 cm.[2,3]
- The Comparison of Surveillance Versus Aortic Endografting for Small Aneurysm Repair (CAESAR) trial randomized 360 patients to surveillance or EVAR and showed that mortality and rupture rates in AAAs <5.5 cm are low and no clear advantage was shown with an early EVAR strategy.[4]
- The SVS practice guidelines on the care of patients with an abdominal aortic aneurysm recommend elective repair for patients at low or acceptable surgical risk with a fusiform AAA >5.5 cm.[5]

Summary and Implications: Patients with a small AAA (4–5 cm in diameter) did not benefit from early EVAR. Rigorous surveillance with selective aneurysm treatment is a safe management option for this cohort of patients due to the low risk of rupture.

CLINICAL CASE: 70-YEAR-OLD PATIENT WITH SMALL AAA

Case History

A 70-year-old female patient is found to have an incidental finding of a 4.2-cm AAA on an ultrasound scan obtained for gallstone disease. She suffers from hypothyroidism and diabetes and stopped smoking 5 years ago. She presents to your clinic for your opinion on the management of her AAA. Based on the current evidence, should the patient undergo surgical repair?

Suggested Answer

The PIVOTAL study showed no survival benefit from early EVAR despite a very low perioperative mortality. Therefore, she should be entered into a surveillance program until the aneurysm reaches treatment threshold or unless it expands rapidly (1 cm in 1 year) or becomes symptomatic.

References

1. Ouriel K, Clair DG, Kent KC, Zarins CK. Endovascular repair compared with surveillance for patients with small abdominal aortic aneurysms. *J Vasc Surg.* 201051(5):1081–1087.
2. Lederle FA, Wilson SE, Johnson GR, et al. Immediate repair compared with surveillance of small abdominal aortic aneurysms. *N Engl J Med.* 2002;346(19):1437–1444.
3. United Kingdom Small Aneurysm Trial Participants. Long-term outcomes of immediate repair compared with surveillance of small abdominal aortic aneurysm. *N Engl J Med.* 2002;346(19):1445–1452.
4. Cao P, De Rango P, Verzini F, et al. Comparison of surveillance versus aortic endografting for small aneurysm repair (CAESAR): Results from a randomised trial. *Eur J Vasc Endovasc Surg.* 2011;41(1):13–25.
5. Chaikof EL, Dalman RL, Eskandari MK, et al. The Society for Vascular Surgery practice guidelines on the care of patients with an abdominal aortic aneurysm. *J Vasc Surg.* 2018;67(1):2–77.

21

Endovascular Versus Open Repair of Abdominal Aortic Aneurysm in 15 Years' Follow-up of the UK Endovascular Aneurysm Repair Trial 1 (EVAR 1)

A Randomized Controlled Trial

> Despite the operative benefit for the EVAR group with lower aneurysm and total mortality after 6 months, this benefit was lost partly due to secondary rupture and aneurysm-related causes of death.
>
> THE EVAR 1 INVESTIGATORS

Research Question: How does endovascular repair of abdominal aortic aneurysm (AAA) compare with open repair in patients judged to be fit for both procedures?[1]

Funding: UK National Institute for Health Research and Camelia Botnar Arterial Research Foundation

Year Study Began: 1999

Year Study Published: 2016

Study Location: 37 clinical centers from the UK

Who Was Studied: Patients aged ≥60 years were included if (1) they had an aortic aneurysm of ≥5.5 cm in diameter (assessed with computed tomography [CT]), with aortic morphology compatible with endograft placement within the manufacturers' instructions for use and (w) they were deemed fit for open repair with an acceptable risk of postoperative death for either procedure.

Who Was Excluded: Patients were excluded if (1) their aneurysm was anatomically unsuitable for an endovascular aneurysm repair (EVAR) device, (2) their AAA was <5.5 cm in diameter, or (3) they refused to enter into the trial or refused to receive a CT scan or further treatment.

Patients: 1,252

Study Overview

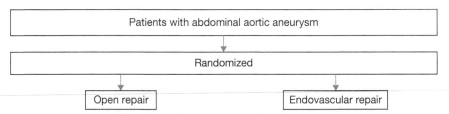

Figure 21.1 Design of EVAR 1 randomized controlled trial

Study Intervention: Patients were randomly assigned to open or endovascular repair. Physicians were encouraged to perform the procedure within 1 month of randomization. Patients were subsequently followed up once a year for clinical and imaging assessment.

Follow-up: Mean follow-up of 12.7 years

Endpoints: Primary outcomes were aneurysm-related mortality and all-cause mortality. Secondary outcomes included reinterventions, time to first reintervention, first reintervention for a life-threatening problem, and first serious re-intervention.

RESULTS

- During the follow-up period, 910 deaths occurred, 101 (11%) of which were aneurysm-related. Overall aneurysm-related mortality was 1.1 deaths per 100 person-years in the EVAR group and 0.9 deaths per 100 person-years in the open repair group (adjusted hazard ratio [HR] 1.31, 95% confidence interval [CI] 0.86–1.99, p = 0.21).

- For all-cause mortality, we recorded 9.3 deaths per 100 person-years in the EVAR group and 8.9 deaths per 100 person-years in the open repair group (adjusted HR 1.11, 95% CI 0.97–1.27, p = 0.14).
- In the early postoperative period (0–6 months), patients in the EVAR group had a lower aneurysm-related and all-cause mortality, but beyond 8 years, open repair had a significantly lower aneurysm-related and all-cause mortality.
- 258 graft-related reinterventions were undertaken in 165 patients in the EVAR group and 105 were done in 74 patients in the open repair group. The reintervention rate was significantly higher in the EVAR group for any reintervention and serious reinterventions than in the open group. There were higher rates of first reintervention as well as life-threatening and serious reintervention in the EVAR group.

Criticisms and Limitations: A limitation of the trial is that the devices were implanted between 1999 and 2004. Since then, techniques and technology have improved and might be expected to produce better results.

The reintervention rate might have been artificially higher in the EVAR group due to type 2 endoleaks being treated; we now know that these are mostly benign and can often be safely monitored without intervention.

Other Relevant Studies and Information

- The Anevrysme de l'aorte abdominale: Chirurgie versus Endoprothese (ACE) trial, a multicenter randomized controlled trial in France comparing open and endovascular AAA repair, showed that in patients with low to intermediate risk factors, open repair of AAA is as safe as EVAR and remains a more durable option.[2]
- UK National Institute for Health and Care Excellence (NICE) AAA guidelines recommend offering open surgical repair for people with unruptured AAAs unless it is contraindicated because of their abdominal co-pathology, anesthetic risks, and/or medical comorbidities and considering EVAR for patients with co-pathology such as a hostile abdomen or stoma.[3]
- The European Society for Vascular Surgery guidelines on the management of abdominal aorto-iliac artery aneurysms recommend EVAR as the preferred treatment modality for most patients with

suitable anatomy and reasonable life expectancy. The guidelines also recommend that in patients with long life expectancy, open AAA repair should be considered as the preferred treatment modality.[4]

Summary and Implications: Compared to an open repair, EVAR has an early survival benefit but inferior late survival. Patients who receive EVAR require life-long surveillance and reintervention if necessary. For this reason, younger and healthier patients might benefit from an open repair to avoid reinterventions.

CLINICAL CASE: ASYMPTOMATIC AAA

Case History
A 65-year-old man presents to your clinic with an AAA measuring 5.5 cm following a screening ultrasound. The patient is asymptomatic and is known to suffer from well-controlled hypertension. He is currently taking aspirin and amlodipine on a daily basis. How would you manage this patient?

Suggested Answer
The patient has been found to have an aneurysm that has already reached treatment threshold. The EVAR 1 trial has shown that EVAR and open surgery have similar long-term survival, with higher reintervention rates with EVAR. In view of the patient being relatively young and medically well, open repair might be more beneficial to decrease long-term complications and reinterventions.

References

1. Patel R, Sweeting MJ, Powell JT, Greenhalgh RM; EVAR trial investigators. Endovascular versus open repair of abdominal aortic aneurysm in 15-years' follow-up of the UK Endovascular Aneurysm Repair trial 1 (EVAR trial 1): A randomised controlled trial. *Lancet.* 2016;388(10058):2366–2374.
2. Becquemin JP, Pillet JC, Lescalie F, et al. A randomized controlled trial of endovascular aneurysm repair versus open surgery for abdominal aortic aneurysms in low- to moderate-risk patients. *J Vasc Surg.* 2011;53(5):1167–1173.
3. National Institute for Health and Care Excellence (NICE). Abdominal aortic aneurysm: Diagnosis and management. 2020. https://www.nice.org.uk/guidance/ng156
4. Wanhainen A, Verzini F, Van Herzeele I, et al. European Society for Vascular Surgery (ESVS) 2019 clinical practice guidelines on the management of abdominal aorto-iliac artery aneurysms. *Eur J Vasc Endovasc Surg.* 2019;57(1):8–93.

22

Endovascular Repair of Abdominal Aortic Aneurysm in Patients Physically Ineligible for Open Repair (EVAR 2)

> The majority of EVAR 2 patients had a limited life expectancy and hence at no time does aneurysm repair confer an overall survival benefit.
>
> THE EVAR 2 INVESTIGATORS

Research Question: How does endovascular repair of abdominal aortic aneurysm (AAA) compare with no intervention in patients judged to be unfit for open repair?[1]

Funding: UK National Institute for Health Research and Camelia Botnar Arterial Research Foundation

Year Study Began: 1999

Year Study Published: 2017

Study Location: 33 clinical centers from the UK

Who Was Studied: Patients aged ≥60 years were included if (1) they had an AAA of ≥5.5 cm in diameter (assessed with computed tomography [CT]) and (2) they were deemed unfit for open repair.

Who Was Excluded: Patients were excluded if (1) the anatomy was unsuitable for EVAR or (2) they refused to consent.

Patients: 404

Study Overview

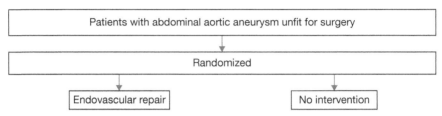

Figure 22.1 Design of EVAR 2 randomized controlled trial

Study Intervention: Patients were randomly assigned to EVAR or no intervention. Physicians were encouraged to perform the procedure within 1 month of randomization in the EVAR group.

Follow-up: Mean follow-up of 4.2 years

Endpoints: The primary outcomes for this trial were all-cause and aneurysm-related mortality. The secondary outcome was the rate of reintervention in each group.

RESULTS

- There were no significant differences in baseline characteristics between the two groups; mean age was 76.8 years and 347 (86%) were men.
- A total of 179 patients in the EVAR group and 71 patients in the no-intervention group underwent repair during follow-up.
- During the entire follow-up period, there were 187 deaths in the EVAR group and 194 in the no-intervention group ($p = 0.52$).
- By 12 years of follow-up, there was no significant difference in life expectancy between the groups (both 4.2 years; $p = 0.97$).
- However, overall aneurysm-related mortality was significantly lower in the EVAR group (27 deaths) compared with the 57 deaths in the no-intervention group ($p = 0.019$).
- 54 graft-related reinterventions were performed in 38 patients in the EVAR group and 21 graft-related reinterventions were performed in 15 patients in the no-intervention group ($p = 0.03$).

Criticisms and Limitations: The main criticism of the study is the significant crossover rate from no intervention to EVAR.

Another limitation is that there was no clear protocol or guideline on how fitness for open surgery was to be judged; the decision was left to the local centers. The lack of standardization limits the ability to produce criteria for which patients are unfit to undergo surgery.

Another limitation is that practice now includes improved devices and epidural anesthesia is more widely used; therefore, patients might have an improved recovery from the procedure.

Other Relevant Studies and Information

- UK National Institute for Health and Care Excellence (NICE) AAA guidelines recommend considering either conservative management or EVAR for those with anesthetic risks and/or medical comorbidities that would contraindicate open repair.[2]
- The European Society for Vascular Surgery guidelines on the management of abdominal aorto-iliac artery aneurysms recommend that for patients with limited life expectancy, elective AAA repair is not recommended.[3]
- The Society for Vascular Surgery practice guidelines on the care of patients with an AAA recommend informing high-risk patients of their Vascular Quality Initiative (VQI) perioperative mortality risk score to help them to make an informed decision about whether proceed with aneurysm repair.[4]

Summary and Implications: In this trial comparing EVAR and conservative management for AAA in patients unfit for open surgery, EVAR did not increase overall life expectancy but reduced aneurysm-related mortality. Patients unfit for open surgery should be advised that there is no survival benefit with EVAR.

CLINICAL CASE: AAA IN A PATIENT UNFIT FOR OPEN REPAIR

Case History

An 86-year-old man is referred to your clinic following an incidental finding of a 5.8-cm AAA. The aneurysm is suitable for EVAR. He suffers from chronic obstructive pulmonary disease (COPD), ischemic heart disease, and hypertension. He mobilizes with a stick and is supported by his daughter at home. How would you manage this patient?

Suggested Answer

This patient requires further preoperative workup. The echocardiogram shows a left ventricular function of 25%, and following an anesthetic review he is declared unfit for open repair. The EVAR 2 trial has shown no survival benefit with EVAR. The outcomes of the trial should be explained to the patient in detail, and you should proceed with conservative management.

References

1. Sweeting MJ, Patel R, Powell JT, Greenhalgh RM; EVAR Trial Investigators. Endovascular repair of abdominal aortic aneurysm in patients physically ineligible for open repair: Very long-term follow-up in the EVAR-2 randomized controlled trial. *Ann Surg.* 2017;266(5):713–719.
2. National Institute for Health and Care Excellence (NICE). Abdominal aortic aneurysm: Diagnosis and management. 2020. https://www.nice.org.uk/guidance/ng156
3. Wanhainen A, Verzini F, Van Herzeele I, et al. European Society for Vascular Surgery (ESVS) 2019 clinical practice guidelines on the management of abdominal aorto-iliac artery aneurysms. *Eur J Vasc Endovasc Surg.* 2019;57(1):8–93.
4. Chaikof EL, Dalman RL, Eskandari MK, et al. The Society for Vascular Surgery practice guidelines on the care of patients with an abdominal aortic aneurysm. *J Vasc Surg.* 2018;67(1):2–77.

23

Open Versus Endovascular Repair of Abdominal Aortic Aneurysm (OVER)

Among younger patients, endovascular repair resulted in somewhat higher long-term overall survival than open repair.

THE OVER INVESTIGATORS

Research Question: What are the long-term results of elective endovascular versus open repair of an abdominal aortic aneurysm (AAA)?[1]

Funding: Department of Veterans Affairs Office of Research and Development

Year Study Began: 2002

Year Study Published: 2019

Study Location: 42 clinical centers from the US

Who Was Studied: Patients were eligible if they had an AAA for which elective repair was planned and were candidates for both endovascular and open repair.

Who Was Excluded: Patients were excluded if (1) their aneurysm was anatomically unsuitable for endovascular repair, (2) their aneurysm was <5 cm in diameter, (3) they refused to enter into the trial, or (4) they were unlikely to adhere to trial requirements.

Patients: 881

Study Overview

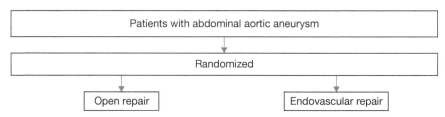

Figure 23.1 Design of OVER randomized controlled trial

Study Intervention: Patients were randomly assigned to open or endovascular repair. The protocol required that the vascular surgeons and interventional radiologists had performed a minimum of 10 previous endovascular and open repair procedures. Aneurysm repair was aimed to be performed within 6 weeks after randomization.

Follow-up: Mean follow-up was 8.4 years.

Endpoints: The primary outcome was all-cause mortality. Secondary outcomes were all-cause mortality as assessed in prespecified subgroups and secondary therapeutic procedures that resulted directly or indirectly from the initial procedure.

RESULTS

- There was no significant difference in the primary outcome of all-cause mortality between the endovascular repair group and the open repair group. A total of 302 deaths occurred in the endovascular repair group and 306 deaths occurred in the open repair group.
- A survival advantage with endovascular repair was seen early: From years 4 through 8, a survival advantage was seen with open repair. However, after 8 years, no difference was observed (p = 0.61).
- There were 12 aneurysm-related deaths (2.7%) in the endovascular repair group and 16 (3.7%) in the open repair group; with two and 11 occurring during the perioperative period, respectively.
- AAA rupture occurred in seven patients (1.6%) in the endovascular repair group and in no patients in the open repair group.
- There were 193 secondary therapeutic procedures involving 117 patients in the endovascular repair group and 116 secondary procedures involving 85 patients in the open repair group (p = 0.04).

Criticisms and Limitations: A limitation of the trial is that devices, imaging software, and hybrid theaters have evolved since the OVER trial. In addition to this, experience of endografts has developed and results for endovascular repair might well have improved since the study.

A large number of patients (n = 382) in the trial had aneurysms <5.5 cm in diameter, for which guidelines generally recommend nonsurgical management.

Other Relevant Studies and Information

- The Dutch Randomized Endovascular Aneurysm Repair (DREAM) trial, a multicenter randomized controlled trial in the Netherlands and Belgium comparing open and endovascular AAA repair, showed no survival difference between patients who underwent open versus endovascular aneurysm repair, despite a continuously increasing number of reinterventions in the endovascular repair group.[2]
- A meta-analysis of individual patient data from the Endovascular Aneurysm Repair 1 (EVAR 1; see Chapter 21), DREAM, OVER, and Anevrysme de l'aorte abdominale: Chirurgie versus Endoprothese (ACE) trials concluded that the early survival advantage in the endovascular repair group erodes over time.[3]
- The Society for Vascular Surgery practice guidelines on the care of patients with an AAA state that endovascular repair has rapidly expanded as the preferred approach for treatment of AAA.[4]

Summary and Implications: In this trial comparing open and endovascular AAA repairs, long-term overall survival was similar among patients despite an early survival advantage with endovascular repair. Patients who underwent endovascular repair required more secondary therapeutic procedures and interventions following the initial procedure compared to those who received an initial open surgical procedure.

CLINICAL CASE: ASYMPTOMATIC AAA IN A 75-YEAR-OLD MAN

Case History

A 75-year-old man presents to your clinic with an AAA measuring 6 cm. He has been on the local surveillance program for the last 5 years. The patient is asymptomatic and is known to suffer from ischemic heart disease and diabetes.

He is currently taking aspirin, atorvastatin, and amlodipine on a daily basis. How would you manage this patient?

Suggested Answer

The patient now has an aneurysm that has reached treatment threshold. A computed tomographic angiogram is obtained and shows the aneurysm is suitable for endovascular repair. The OVER trial has shown that endovascular and open surgery have similar long-term survival, with an early advantage for endovascular repair. In view of the patient's age and comorbidities, he might tolerate an endovascular repair better, but he should be made aware of the higher reintervention rate with it and the need for long-term surveillance.

References

1. Lederle FA, Kyriakides TC, Stroupe KT, et al.. Open versus endovascular repair of abdominal aortic aneurysm. *N Engl J Med.* 2019;380(22):2126–2135.
2. Van Schaik TG, Yeung KK, Verhagen HJ, et al. Long-term survival and secondary procedures after open or endovascular repair of abdominal aortic aneurysms. *J Vasc Surg.* 2017;66(5):1379–1389.
3. Powell JT, Sweeting MJ, Ulug P, et al. Meta-analysis of individual-patient data from EVAR-1, DREAM, OVER and ACE trials comparing outcomes of endovascular or open repair for abdominal aortic aneurysm over 5 years. *Br J Surg.* 2017;104(3):166–178.
4. Chaikof EL, Dalman RL, Eskandari MK, et al. The Society for Vascular Surgery practice guidelines on the care of patients with an abdominal aortic aneurysm. *J Vasc Surg.* 2018;67(1):2–77.

24

Endovascular or Open Repair Strategy for Ruptured Abdominal Aortic Aneurysm

30-Day Outcomes from the Immediate Management of Patients with Rupture: Open Versus Endovascular Repair (IMPROVE) Randomized Trial

Similar overall 30-day mortality was seen with an endovascular strategy (35%) and open surgical repair (37%).

THE IMPROVE INVESTIGATORS

Research Question: For patients with suspected ruptured abdominal aortic aneurysm (AAA), how does endovascular repair (EVAR) compare to open repair with respect to early mortality?[1]

Funding: National Institute of Health Research

Year Study Began: 2009

Year Study Published: 2014

Study Location: 30 vascular centers (29 UK, 1 Canadian)

Who Was Studied: All patients aged >50 years with a clinical diagnosis of ruptured AAA or ruptured aorto-iliac aneurysm, made by a senior trial hospital clinician (either in emergency medicine or vascular surgery), were eligible for inclusion.

Who Was Excluded: Patients were excluded if (1) they had a previous aneurysm repair, rupture of an isolated internal iliac aneurysm, aorto-caval or aorto-enteric fistulas, recent anatomic assessment of the aorta, or a connective tissue disorder or (2) intervention was considered futile.

Patients: 613

Study Overview

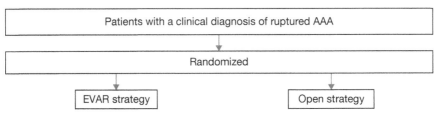

Figure 24.1 Design of IMPROVE randomized controlled trial

Study Intervention: Eligible patients were randomly assigned to an EVAR strategy (immediate computed tomography [CT] followed by EVAR if locally determined as anatomically suitable and open repair when not suitable) or an open strategy with CT being optional.

Follow-up: 30-day follow-up

Endpoints: Primary outcome was 30-day mortality. Secondary outcomes were 24-hour and in-hospital mortality, costs, and time and place of discharge.

RESULTS

- In the EVAR strategy group, 275/316 patients (87%) had a confirmed diagnosis of rupture, eight (3%) had repair of a symptomatic nonruptured aneurysm in the same admission, and 33 (10%) had other discharge diagnoses. Of the patients with ruptured or symptomatic aneurysm, 272 had CT with 174 (64%) considered anatomically suitable for EVAR. EVAR was attempted in 154 patients (four were converted to open repair); open repair was attempted in 112 other patients and 16 patients died before aneurysm repair; and one patient with a symptomatic aneurysm refused repair.
- In the open strategy group, 261/297 patients (88%) had a confirmed diagnosis of rupture, 14 (5%) had repair of a symptomatic intact aneurysm in the same admission, and 22 (7%) had other discharge diagnoses. EVAR was attempted in 36 (13%) patients and open repair in 220 (80%) patients and 19 patients died before aneurysm repair.

- Overall 30-day mortality was not significantly different at 35.4% (112/316) in the EVAR strategy group and 37.4% (111/297) in the open repair group (p = 0.62). Similarly, 30-day mortality was not significantly different between the two groups in those patients with confirmed AAA rupture who received repair (p = 0.31).
- 24-hour and in-hospital mortality rates were not significantly different between the two groups. Hospital stay was shorter in the EVAR group and more patients were also directly discharged home in that group (p < 0.001). However, the average hospital costs within the first 30 days of randomization were similar between the randomized groups.

Criticisms and Limitations: In the trial, the clinical diagnosis of rupture was incorrect in 13% of patients, which was higher than predicted (5%), illustrating the difficulty in making a clinical diagnosis of ruptured aneurysm.

The suitability of ruptured aneurysm for EVAR is subjective and will be defined by the aortic morphology, the experience of the surgeon, and the anesthetic techniques available. This study was intended to examine the role of EVAR strategy and should not be used to promote an EVAR policy for all patients.

Other Relevant Studies and Information

- A Dutch randomized controlled trial randomized patients with ruptured AAA who were fit for both open repair and EVAR and did not show a significant difference in combined death and severe complications between EVAR and open surgery.[2]
- UK National Institute for Health and Care Excellence (NICE) abdominal aortic guidelines recommend considering EVAR or open surgical repair for people with a ruptured AAA; the guidelines also conclude that EVAR provides more benefit than open surgical repair for most people.[3]
- The European Society for Vascular Surgery guidelines on the management of abdominal aorto-iliac artery aneurysms recommend EVAR as the first option for patients with a ruptured AAA.[4]
- The Society for Vascular Surgery practice guidelines on the care of patients with an abdominal aortic aneurysm recommend EVAR over open repair if anatomically feasible.[5]

Summary and Implications: A strategy of EVAR was not associated with significant reduction in either 30-day mortality or cost when compared to an open strategy. Importantly, this trial proved that it was safe to assess patients with suspected rupture with imaging prior to surgical intervention. Most guidelines recommend EVAR as the preferred option if anatomically suitable as it is a less invasive procedure.

CLINICAL CASE: MANAGEMENT OF RUPTURED AAA

Case History

A 64-year-old woman presents to the emergency department following a collapse at home. She was found hypotensive and tachycardic by the paramedics. Following a bolus of fluid in the ambulance, her blood pressure has slightly improved and she is talking on arrival complaining of abdominal pain. On examination, she has a pulsatile mass and a clinical diagnosis of AAA is made. How should she then be managed?

Suggested Answer

She is managed with permissive hypotension with limited fluid resuscitation. The IMPROVE trial showed that a patient with a suspected AAA can be safely managed with an endovascular strategy with an initial CT angiogram. She undergoes a CT angiogram of her whole aorta, which shows a AAA suitable for EVAR. She is taken to the hybrid theater and under local anesthesia she undergoes an endovascular repair of her AAA. Following an initially slow recovery, she is discharged home on day 7.

References

1. IMPROVE Trial Investigators. Endovascular or open repair strategy for ruptured abdominal aortic aneurysm: 30-day outcomes from IMPROVE randomised trial. *BMJ*. 2014;348:f7661.
2. Reimerink JJ, Hoornweg LL, Vahl AC, et al. Endovascular repair versus open repair of ruptured abdominal aortic aneurysms: A multicenter randomized controlled trial. *Ann Surg*. 2013;258:248–256.
3. National Institute for Health and Care Excellence (NICE). Abdominal aortic aneurysm: Diagnosis and management. 2020. https://www.nice.org.uk/guidance/ng156
4. Wanhainen A, Verzini F, Van Herzeele I, et al. European Society for Vascular Surgery (ESVS) 2019 clinical practice guidelines on the management of abdominal aorto-iliac artery aneurysms. *Eur J Vasc Endovasc Surg*. 2019;57(1):8–93.
5. Chaikof EL, Dalman RL, Eskandari MK, et al. The Society for Vascular Surgery practice guidelines on the care of patients with an abdominal aortic aneurysm. *J Vasc Surg*. 2018;67(1):2–77.

25

Meta-analysis of Fenestrated Endovascular Aneurysm Repair Versus Open Surgical Repair of Juxtarenal Abdominal Aortic Aneurysms

> Long-term survival was similar for [open surgical repair] and [fenestrated endovascular repair] in this meta-analysis.
>
> JONES ET AL.

Research Question: What are the short- and long-term outcomes of fenestrated endovascular repair (FEVAR) and open surgical repair (OSR) for the management of juxtarenal abdominal aortic aneurysms (AAAs)?[1]

Funding: None

Year Range for Searches: 2007–2017

Year Study Published: 2019

Number of Studies Included in Systematic Review: 27 studies included in the meta-analysis

Which Studies Were Included: Prospective and retrospective cohort studies, as well as case series involving >20 patients undergoing elective complex aneurysm repair, published from 2007 onwards were included.

Which Studies Were Excluded: Registry data were excluded to avoid duplication of data. Studies were excluded if presenting data for thoracoabdominal
aortic aneurysms, ruptures, surgeon-modified grafts, chimney/snorkel repairs,
and branched devices.

Patients: 2,975

Study Overview: This was a meta-analysis of FEVAR versus OSR of juxtarenal
AAA. A comprehensive search strategy of the English literature was used to include the following terms: fenestrated endovascular repair, aneurysm, open repair, and juxtarenal aneurysm.

Follow-up: Follow-up ranged from 1 to 67 months.

Endpoints: The primary outcomes were 30-day/in-hospital mortality and postoperative renal insufficiency. Secondary outcomes included major complication
rates, postoperative permanent dialysis, rate of reintervention, long-term survival, and rates of endoleak.

RESULTS

- A total of 2,975 patients were included: 1,476 underwent FEVAR and
  1,499 underwent OSR. Patients undergoing FEVAR had more medical
  comorbidities. Preexisting renal dysfunction was twice as high in the
  FEVAR cohort; these patients also displayed higher rates of ischemic heart
  disease and pulmonary dysfunction (Table 25.1).

Table 25.1 SUMMARY OF BASELINE CHARACTERISTICS

	FEVAR	OSR
Age (years)	73.2	72.1
Aneurysm diameter (cm)	6.1	6.3
Renal dysfunction (%)	37.8	16.7
Ischemic heart disease (%)	54.5	49.5
Pulmonary dysfunction (%)	39.4	31.9
Diabetes (%)	17.7	13.7

- The pooled rate of early postoperative mortality following FEVAR was not
  significantly different at 3.3% versus 4.2% after OSR. Estimated long-term
  survival was similar for FEVAR and OSR.

- The pooled rate of postoperative renal insufficiency was not significantly different between FEVAR (16.2%, 95% confidence interval [CI] 10.4–23.0) and OSR (23.8%, 95% CI 15.2–33.6). The pooled rate of permanent dialysis was 0.8% (0.4–1.4%) and 1.7% (1.0–2.5%), respectively.
- The major early complication rate was higher after OSR at 43.5% (34.4–52.8%) than FEVAR at 23.1% (16.8–30.1%). Conversely, the rate of late reintervention after FEVAR was higher than that after OSR: 11.1% (6.7–16.4%) versus 2.0% (0.6–4.3%), respectively.

Criticisms and Limitations: The main limitation of this study is that it was not a randomized controlled trial, which means that the two populations are likely to be different with respect to factors such as comorbidities and surgical fitness; as a result, confounding factors may have biased the results.

Other Relevant Studies and Information

- A single-center cohort study from the UK reporting on 173 patients concluded that FEVAR technology for juxtarenal aneurysm repair is safe, with adequate long-term results; however, significant reinterventions are required.[2]
- UK National Institute for Health and Care Excellence (NICE) AAA guidelines recommend that if OSR and FEVAR are both suitable options, complex EVAR should be considered only following a discussion with the patient informing them of its risks compared with the risks of OSR and the uncertainties around whether complex EVAR improves perioperative survival or long-term outcomes when compared with OSR.[3]
- The European Society for Vascular Surgery guidelines on the management of abdominal aorto-iliac artery aneurysms recommend that in complex EVAR of juxtarenal AAA, EVAR with fenestrated stent-grafts should be considered the preferred treatment option when feasible rather than OSR.[4]

Summary and Implications: In this meta-analysis comparing outcomes in patients with juxtarenal AAA undergoing either open or endovascular repair, there was no significant difference in 30-day mortality; however, FEVAR was associated with significantly lower morbidity than OSR. Long-term durability is a concern, with far higher reintervention rates after FEVAR. Patients who undergo this procedure need to be aware of the need for life-long surveillance.

CLINICAL CASE: A 72-YEAR-OLD MAN WITH A JUXTARENAL ANEURYSM

Case History

A 72-year-old man is referred to your clinic with an asymptomatic 6.3-cm juxtarenal aneurysm. He is known to suffer from ischemic heart disease and hypertension. He lives independently at home with his wife. How would you manage this patient?

Suggested Answer

This patient has an aneurysm that has reached threshold for repair. A computed tomographic angiogram is obtained to define the anatomy further and confirms that a fenestrated repair is possible. The patient needs to be counseled about the benefits and risks of open and endovascular repair in detail. The meta-analysis has shown lower morbidity with FEVAR, but the patient needs to be told about the long-term higher reintervention rate.

References

1. Jones AD, Waduud MA, Walker P, et al. Meta-analysis of fenestrated endovascular aneurysm repair versus open surgical repair of juxtarenal abdominal aortic aneurysms over the last 10 years. *BJS Open*. 2019;3(5):572–584.
2. Roy IN, Millen AM, Jones SM, et al. Long-term follow-up of fenestrated endovascular repair for juxtarenal aortic aneurysm. *Br J Surg*. 2017;104(8):1020–1027.
3. National Institute for Health and Care Excellence (NICE). Abdominal aortic aneurysm: Diagnosis and management. 2020. https://www.nice.org.uk/guidance/ng156
4. Wanhainen A, Verzini F, Van Herzeele I, et al. European Society for Vascular Surgery (ESVS) 2019 clinical practice guidelines on the management of abdominal aorto-iliac artery aneurysms. *Eur J Vasc Endovasc Surg*. 2019;57(1):8–93.

Visceral and Renal Arterial Disease

JULIEN AL SHAKARCHI AND RICHARD DOWNING

26

Stenting and Medical Therapy for Atherosclerotic Renal Artery Stenosis

The Cardiovascular Outcomes in Renal Atherosclerotic Lesion (CORAL) Trial

> Renal artery stenting did not confer a significant benefit with respect to the prevention of clinical events when added to comprehensive, multifactorial medical therapy in people with atherosclerotic renal-artery stenosis and hypertension or chronic kidney disease.
>
> THE CORAL INVESTIGATORS

Research Question: For patients with renal artery stenosis, what are the effects of renal artery stenting on the incidence of major adverse cardiovascular and renal events?[1]

Funding: National Heart, Lung, and Blood Institute. Medications were donated by AstraZeneca and Pfizer.

Year Study Began: 2005

Year Study Published: 2014

Study Location: 112 clinical centers from 10 countries

Who Was Studied: Adult patients with severe renal artery stenosis were eligible if they had either (1) hypertension with a systolic blood pressure of ≥155 mmHg

while receiving two or more antihypertensive medications or (2) renal dysfunction (defined as stage 3 or greater chronic kidney disease [CKD]).

Who Was Excluded: Exclusion criteria were renal artery stenosis due to
fibromuscular dysplasia, CKD from a cause other than ischemic nephropathy,
kidney length of <7 cm, and a lesion that could not be treated with the use of a
single stent.

Patients: 947

Study Overview

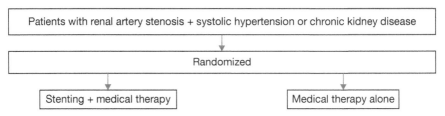

Figure 26.1 Design of CORAL randomized controlled trial

Study Intervention: Patients were randomly assigned to either medical therapy
alone or stenting plus medical therapy. The protocol for medical treatment was
candesartan with or without hydrochlorothiazide and amlodipine combined
with atorvastatin.

Follow-up: Median follow-up was 43 months.

Endpoints: *Primary outcome:* Major cardiovascular or renal event (a composite
of death from cardiovascular or renal causes, stroke, myocardial infarction, hos-
pitalization for congestive heart failure, progressive renal insufficiency, or the
need for permanent renal-replacement therapy). *Secondary outcomes:* Individual
components of the composite primary outcome and all-cause mortality.

RESULTS

- The mean age of patients was 69 years, with an equal gender distribution.
- 19 of the 472 patients randomized to medical therapy crossed over to
  stenting (4%). Stents were placed in 434 of the 459 patients randomized
  to stenting (94.6%).

- There was no significant difference in the occurrence of the primary composite endpoint between the stent group and medical therapy group (35.1% and 35.8%, p = 0.58) (Table 26.1).
- There was also no significant difference between the two groups in the rates of the components of the primary outcome measure or all-cause mortality.
- At baseline, participants were taking a mean of 2.1 antihypertensive medications. At the end of the study, the number of medications increased in both the stent group and the medical therapy group but did not differ significantly between the two groups (3.3 and 3.5 medications, respectively; p = 0.24). Systolic blood pressure declined in both the medical therapy group (by 15.6 mmHg) and the stent group (by 16.6 mmHg).
- Subgroup analyses showed no difference in the primary outcomes for creatinine level, glomerular filtration rate (GFR), diabetes, sex, global ischemia, race, baseline systolic blood pressure, age, geographic location, and maximal diameter of the stenosis.

Table 26.1 CLINICAL ENDPOINTS FOR BOTH GROUPS

Endpoint	Stenting + medical therapy group (n = 459)	Medical therapy group (n = 472)	Hazard ratio (95% CI)	p value
Major cardiovascular or renal event	161 (35.1%)	169 (35.8%)	0.94 (0.76–1.17)	0.58
Death from any cause	63 (13.7%)	76 (16.1%)	0.80 (0.58–1.12)	0.20
Death from cardiovascular causes	41 (8.9%)	45 (9.5%)	0.89 (0.58–1.36)	0.60
Death from renal causes	2 (0.4%)	1 (0.2%)	1.89 (0.17–20.85)	0.60
Stroke	16 (3.5%)	23 (4.9%)	0.68 (0.36–1.28)	0.23
Myocardial infarction	40 (8.7%)	37 (7.8%)	1.09 (0.70–1.71)	0.70
Hospitalization for congestive heart failure	39 (8.5%)	39 (8.3%)	1.00 (0.64–1.56)	0.99
Progressive renal insufficiency	77 (16.8%)	89 (18.9%)	0.86 (0.64–1.17)	0.34
Permanent renal-replacement therapy	16 (3.5%)	8 (1.7%)	1.98 (0.85–4.62)	0.11

CI, confidence interval.

Criticisms and Limitations: One criticism of this randomized controlled trial (RCT) is that patients with renal artery stenosis of ≥60% were included. The mean percent stenosis in the stenting and medical groups was 67.3% and 66.9%, respectively. There is debate about the severity of stenosis that is necessary to justify intervention, and a higher degree of stenosis (>80%) might have been a more appropriate cutoff to use for trial inclusion.

As with any RCT, some patients who were screened and deemed to be eligible were not enrolled in the trial due to physician preference, limiting the generalizability of the findings to real-world settings.

Changes were also made to the enrollment criteria during the trial; for instance, the threshold for defining systolic hypertension (155 mmHg) was abandoned.

Other Relevant Studies and Information

- The Angioplasty and Stenting for Renal Artery Lesions (ASTRAL) study randomized 806 patients with atherosclerotic renovascular disease to either revascularization or medical therapy only. It found substantial risks but no evidence of a worthwhile clinical benefit from revascularization.[2]
- Another RCT showed that stent placement with medical treatment had no clear effect on progression of renal disease but led to a small number of significant procedure-related complications.[3]
- The 2017 European Society of Cardiology (ESC) guidelines on the diagnosis and treatment of peripheral arterial diseases, in collaboration with the European Society for Vascular Surgery (ESVS), indicate that routine revascularization is not recommended for atherosclerotic renal artery stenosis.[4]

Summary and Implications: In this RCT comparing renal artery stenting versus medical management for patients with atherosclerotic renal artery stenosis, renal artery stenting did not confer a significant benefit with respect to the prevention of clinical events.

CLINICAL CASE: RENAL ARTERY STENOSIS

Case History

One of your cardiology colleagues seeks your opinion on one of his challenging patients. Despite being on three antihypertensive medications, his patient is still hypertensive, with a systolic pressure of 170 mmHg. The patient is a 65-year-old man with a previous history of ischemic heart disease and stage

2 CKD. An ultrasound duplex has shown a unilateral 90% renal artery stenosis. How would you manage this patient?

Suggested Answer

The CORAL study has shown that patients with renal artery stenosis do not benefit from stenting in terms of preventing cardiac and renal events. In addition to this, the ASTRAL study did not show any benefit for such patients. In view of this evidence, the patient should be managed medically with multifactorial antihypertensive therapy.

References

1. Cooper CJ, Murphy TP, Cutlip DE, et al. Stenting and medical therapy for atherosclerotic renal-artery stenosis. *N Engl J Med.* 2014;370(1):13–22.
2. The ASTRAL Investigators. Revascularization versus medical therapy for renal-artery stenosis. *N Engl J Med.* 2009;361:1953–1962.
3. Bax L, Woittiez AJ, Kouwenberg HJ, et al. Stent placement in patients with atherosclerotic renal artery stenosis and impaired renal function: A randomized trial. *Ann Intern Med.* 2009;150:840–848.
4. Aboyans V, Ricco JB, Bartelink MEL, et al. 2017 ESC guidelines on the diagnosis and treatment of peripheral arterial diseases, in collaboration with the European Society for Vascular Surgery (ESVS): Document covering atherosclerotic disease of extracranial carotid and vertebral, mesenteric, renal, upper and lower extremity arteries. *Eur Heart J.* 2018;39(9):763–816.

Patient Survival After Open and Endovascular Mesenteric Revascularization for Chronic Mesenteric Ischemia

> The choice of treatment is based on patient comorbidities, physician preference, and experience at the institution.
>
> TALLARITA ET AL.

Research Question: What are long-term patient survival and causes of death after open (OR) versus endovascular (ER) mesenteric revascularization for atherosclerotic chronic mesenteric ischemia (CMI)?[1]

Funding: None

Years Patients Were Treated: 1991–2010

Year Study Published: 2013

Number of Patients: 343

Who Was Studied: A diagnosis of CMI was made in patients who had classic symptoms (abdominal pain, postprandial pain, weight loss, and "food fear") for >2 weeks and angiographic evidence of high-grade stenosis or occlusion of at least one mesenteric artery.

Who Was Excluded: Patients with acute or acute-on-chronic mesenteric ischemia, asymptomatic lesions, vasculitis, median arcuate ligament syndrome, or other non-atherosclerotic etiologies were excluded.

Study Overview: An analysis of retrospective data was done to identify all adult patients who had been diagnosed with CMI between 1991 and 2010. Outcomes were compared between patients receiving open versus endovascular treatment of atherosclerotic lesions.

Follow-up: Median follow-up was 96 months.

Endpoints: The primary endpoint was patient survival at 5 years. The secondary end point was freedom from mesenteric-related death.

RESULTS

- 343 patients with CMI with a mean age of 68 years were treated with either OR (n = 187) or ER (n = 156). 256 patients of the patients (75%) were women.
- There were a disproportionate number of intermediate-risk and high-risk patients in the ER group, predominantly as a consequence of cardiac, respiratory, and renal disease.
- In the OR group there were five procedure-related deaths from myocardial infarction (n = 2), mesenteric ischemia (n = 2), and respiratory failure (n = 1). In the ER group, there were four deaths from bowel ischemia secondary to embolization (n = 2) and myocardial Infarction (n = 2).
- There were no significant differences in rates of reinterventions for recurrent symptoms or a high-grade restenosis between the OR (14%) and ER (21%) groups. Overall, 10 OR patients (5.8%) and six ER patients (4.1%) died of late mesenteric-related causes.
- For the entire cohort, the combined rate of early and late mesenteric-related death was 8% for the OR group and 6.4% for the ER group. The overall 5-year patient survival was 69% in the OR group and 44% in the ER group (p < 0.001), reflecting the greater comorbidity of patients in the latter group. However, freedom from mesenteric-related death was not significantly different between the OR group (91%) and the ER group (91%) during the follow-up period.

Criticisms and Limitations: First, and most importantly, this was an observational study, and thus confounding factors may have biased the results. For example, patients in the ER group were disproportionately likely to have cardiac, respiratory, and renal disease, which likely led to poorer outcomes in those assigned to ER. A randomized trial design would be necessary to more rigorously compare the two treatment approaches.

During the two decades of the study, there has been significant progress in best medical therapy, surgical techniques, and endovascular technology, which may affect treatment outcomes. Thus, findings from this analysis may not be generalizable to the current era.

Other Relevant Studies and Information

• The Society for Vascular Surgery clinical practice guidelines for chronic mesenteric ischemia state that ER with a balloon-expandable covered intraluminal stent is the recommended initial treatment for CMI, with OR reserved for select younger patients and those who are not candidates for endovascular treatment due to their vascular anatomy.[2]
• The European Society for Vascular Surgery guidelines indicate that in patients with CMI needing revascularization, the superior long-term results of open surgery must be offset against a possible early benefit of endovascular intervention with regard to periprocedural mortality and morbidity.[3]

Summary and Implications: In this observational analysis comparing outcomes of patients with CMI treated with either ER or OR, long-term patient survival was nearly identical. A randomized trial would be required to more rigorously compare these two management strategies.

CLINICAL CASE: CMI

Case History
A 58-year-old female patient presents with abdominal pain and weight loss. She is initially admitted under the general surgeons, who ask for a vascular opinion. On review, you establish that she has suffered from postprandial pain

for >6 months and has fear of eating as a result. She has lost nearly 10 kg during the same time period. How would you manage this patient?

Suggested Answer

I would review her investigations, as she has previously been assessed by multiple health care professionals. The results of gastroscopy and colonoscopy ordered by her family doctor were normal. The computed tomographic (CT) scan of her abdomen obtained during this admission revealed possible mesenteric arterial disease but no other abnormality. You order a formal CT angiogram of her aorta, which confirms an occluded celiac artery, a tight stenosis of the superior mesenteric artery, and a small-caliber patent inferior mesenteric artery. Following a multidisciplinary meeting and extensive counseling, she undergoes successful superior mesenteric artery stenting, with resolution of her symptoms and subsequent weight gain.

References

1. Tallarita T, Oderich GS, Gloviczki P, et al. Patient survival after open and endovascular mesenteric revascularization for chronic mesenteric ischemia. *J Vasc Surg.* 2013;57(3):747–755.
2. Huber TS, Björck M, Chandra A, et al. Chronic mesenteric ischemia: Clinical practice guidelines from the Society for Vascular Surgery. *J Vasc Surg.* 2021;73(1S):87S–115S.
3. Björck M, Koelemay M, Acosta S, et al. Management of the diseases of mesenteric arteries and veins: Clinical practice guidelines of the European Society of Vascular Surgery (ESVS). *Eur J Vasc Endovasc Surg.* 2017;53(4):460–510.

28

Splenic Artery Aneurysms

Two Decades of Experience at the Mayo Clinic

> Most splenic artery aneurysms remain relatively small and rarely enlarge, become symptomatic, or rupture.
>
> ABBAS ET AL.

Research Question: What is the natural history of splenic artery aneurysms (SAAs) and outcomes of treatment?[1]

Funding: None

Years Patients Were Treated: 1980–1998

Year Study Published: 2002

Number of Patients: 217

Who Was Studied: Patients with SAAs diagnosed by imaging studies, surgical exploration, or autopsy evaluation.

Who Was Excluded: Patients with splenic artery pseudo-aneurysms were excluded.

Study Overview: Analysis of retrospective data to identify all adult patients who had been diagnosed with SAA between 1980 and 1998.

Follow-up: Mean follow-up was 70 and 89 months in the operated non-ruptured and ruptured groups, respectively, and 75 months in the non-operated group.

Endpoints: The records were analyzed with regard to demographics, comorbidities, clinical presentation, aneurysm characteristics, imaging studies, management (including operative intervention), and outcome.

RESULTS

- 217 patients were found to have SAA. 171 of them were female (78.8%), and the majority of them (96%) were white. Mean age at presentation was 61.7 years. Only 10 patients presented with rupture (4.6%); four were symptomatic and not ruptured (1.8%), and 203 were asymptomatic (93.6%). The mean SAA diameter was 3.1 cm (range 2.3–5 cm) in patients who presented with rupture. In contrast, the mean diameter of non-ruptured SAA was 2.3 cm (range 0.8–5 cm) (Table 28.1).

Table 28.1 ANEURYSM CHARACTERISTICS

Feature	Ruptured aneurysms (n = 10)	Non-ruptured aneurysms (n = 207)
Single aneurysm	10 (100%)	188 (90.7%)
Presence of calcification	9 (90%)	175 (84.5%)
Mean diameter (cm)	3.1	2.3
Range of diameter (cm)	2.3–5	0.8–5

- Non-splenic visceral artery aneurysms were found in only 3.3% of patients. Renal artery aneurysms were the most common non-visceral aneurysm (7.4%).
- 49 patients underwent surgical interventions (22.6%); 10 had emergency procedures because of SAA rupture and 39 patients underwent elective operations. All emergency patients were managed with splenectomy. Ligation of the aneurysm was the most common operation in the elective group (23 patients, 59%), followed by splenectomy (11 patients, 28%) and embolization (five patients, 13%). Operative mortality was 20% and 5.1% in the ruptured and elective groups, respectively. In the elective group, the two deaths were caused by a gastroesophageal anastomotic leak after concomitant gastric resection of carcinoma and by a postoperative myocardial infarction.

- Nonoperative management was chosen in 168 patients (77.4%). Mean aneurysm growth was found to be 0.06 cm/year. No ruptures or other complications related to the aneurysm occurred in any patient during the follow-up period.

Criticisms and Limitations: Because this was an observational study, it is not possible to rigorously compare the relative benefits and risks of different management strategies.

Due to the small size of the analysis, no firm conclusions can be drawn with regard to features of ruptured versus non-ruptured aneurysms. However, calcification does not appear to confer protection against rupture as reported in other publications.

Endovascular management of SAAs has evolved greatly over the last decade, and in most units it has become the mainstay of treatment once size threshold has been reached. Outcomes with these newer management strategies may be different than those reported in this analysis.

Other Relevant Studies and Information

- A systematic review on management options for SAA concluded that endovascular treatment had better short-term results compared with open surgery, including significantly lower perioperative mortality. However, open surgery was associated with fewer late complications and fewer reinterventions during follow-up.[2]
- The Society for Vascular Surgery guidelines on the management of visceral aneurysms recommend treating unruptured true splenic artery aneurysms (TSAAs) of any size in women of childbearing age because of the risk of rupture and unruptured TSAAs >3 cm with a demonstrable increase in size or with associated symptoms. Surveillance was advocated for small (<3 cm), stable asymptomatic TSAAs or those in patients with significant medical comorbidities or limited life expectancy.[3]

Summary and Implications: This analysis of SAAs found that they are rarely symptomatic and enlarge slowly; significant growth is rare. Selective operative management of SAAs is associated with excellent outcomes. Guidelines from major surgical societies recommend consideration of open ligation or transcatheter embolization in patients with symptomatic aneurysms, aneurysms >3 cm, and any SAA in women of childbearing age.

CLINICAL CASE: SAA

Case History

A 72-year-old male is referred to your clinic following an incidental finding of a 1.9-cm calcified splenic artery aneurysm on a computed tomography (CT) scan ordered for nonspecific abdominal pain that had now completely resolved. He suffers from heart failure and stage 3 chronic kidney disease and his BMI is 33. How would you manage this patient?

Suggested Answer

This patient is asymptomatic and the SAA has not reached size threshold for intervention. On reviewing his previous imaging at your institution, he had a previous CT scan from 6 years ago showing a 1.8-cm SAA. You explain to the patients the findings of the scan and reassure him he does not require treatment at present. You order an ultrasound, which identifies the SAA; therefore, you recommend this imaging modality for 2 yearly surveillance scan. After 8 years of follow-up, his aneurysm has not enlarged. Due to his worsening heart failure and in agreement with the patient, you discharge him from surveillance.

References

1. Abbas MA, Stone WM, Fowl RJ, et al. Splenic artery aneurysms: Two decades experience at Mayo Clinic. *Ann Vasc Surg.* 2002;16(4):442–449.
2. Hogendoorn W, Lavida A, Hunink MG, et al. Open repair, endovascular repair, and conservative management of true splenic artery aneurysms. *J Vasc Surg.* 2014;60(6):1667–1676.
3. Chaer RA, Abularrage CJ, Coleman DM, et al. The Society for Vascular Surgery clinical practice guidelines on the management of visceral aneurysm. *J Vasc Surg.* 2020l;72(1S):3S–39S.

29

Renal Artery Aneurysms

A 35-Year Clinical Experience with 252 Aneurysms in 168 Patients

The present series documents the safety, efficacy, and durability of surgical therapy for [renal artery aneurysms].

HENKE ET AL.

Research Question: What is the optimal management for renal artery aneurysms
(RAAs)?[1]

Funding: None

Years Patients Were Treated: 1965–2000

Year Study Published: 2001

Number of Patients: 168 (252 RAAs)

Who Was Studied: Patients with asymptomatic or symptomatic RAA diagnosed on plain abdominal radiographs, intravenous pyelography, computed tomography scan, arteriography, and magnetic resonance angiography.

Who Was Excluded: RAAs associated with trauma, dissections, and connective
diseases such as polyarteritis nodosa were excluded from this analysis.

Study Overview: Analysis of retrospective data to identify all adult patients who had been diagnosed with RAA between 1965 and 2000 in this single large arterial center.

Follow-up: Mean follow-up was 91 months.

Endpoints: Records were extracted for demographics, comorbidities, clinical presentation, aneurysm characteristics, imaging studies, management including operative intervention, and outcome.

RESULTS

- The mean patient age was 51 years (range 13–78), with a female to male ratio of 107:61.
- Most patients had RAAs discovered incidentally because most were asymptomatic. Most common symptoms were pain presumed related to their aneurysm in 29 patients and hematuria in 14 patients. Three patients presented with acute overt RAA rupture.
- Surgical therapy was undertaken in 121 patients with 168 RAAs. 96 patients underwent renal artery reconstructions with an aneurysmectomy and 25 patients underwent planned nephrectomy. Secondary nephrectomy was performed for early surgical failure in eight patients.
- Perioperative complications included postoperative hemorrhage requiring reoperation (n = 1), deep venous thrombosis (n = 1), pneumonia requiring reintubation (n = 1), third-degree heart block (n = 1), and postoperative pancreatitis (n = 1). There were no perioperative deaths, and only one patient had postoperative renal failure requiring hemodialysis.
- Reinterventions were required for seven patients, including percutaneous anastomotic angioplasty (n = 4), early reoperation for graft thrombosis (n = 1), revision of a bypass venous graft for aneurysmal change 23 years after surgery (n = 1), and percutaneous embolization for a stenotic segmental branch causing renovascular hypertension (n = 1).
- There were 86 RAAs involving 61 patients managed with observation alone. The mean RAA size in those observed was nonsignificantly smaller than in the surgical group (1.3 vs. 1.5 cm) with similar location. None of these RAAs were symptomatic. After an average follow-up of 72 months, no RAA ruptures among the nonoperative cases were documented.

Criticisms and Limitations: Because this was an observational study, it is not possible to rigorously compare the relative benefits and risks of different management strategies.

Long-term follow-up data were not available for 14% of patients in the analysis.

Other Relevant Studies and Information

- Endovascular therapy has been found to be an effective and safe primary therapy for RAA; however, long-term follow-up is still lacking.[2]
- The Society for Vascular Surgery guidelines recommend that in patients with uncomplicated RAA of acceptable operative risk, aneurysms >3 cm should be treated with open surgical reconstructive techniques. The guidelines also suggest that endovascular techniques, including stent-graft exclusion of main RAAs, should be reserved for patients with poor operative risk.[3]

Summary and Implications: Surgical therapy of RAAs in selected patients provides excellent long-term clinical outcomes and is often associated with decreased blood pressure. Nonsurgical management was also associated with excellent outcomes.

CLINICAL CASE: RAA

Case History

A 51-year-old woman is found to have a 1.9-cm left RAA on ultrasound. The scan was requested by her physician due to her history of hypertension. She is otherwise medically well and does not suffer from any major comorbidities. How would you manage this patient?

Suggested Answer

This patient is currently asymptomatic and has not met the size threshold for treatment. I would check that the patient is postmenopausal; she confirms that she had her last period 9 years ago. I would put her on a yearly ultrasound surveillance. After 8 years of surveillance, her aneurysm has reached 3 cm in diameter and is suitable for both open and endovascular treatment. She opts for open surgery and makes a good postoperative recovery.

References

1. Henke PK, Cardneau JD, Welling TH 3rd, et al. Renal artery aneurysms: A 35-year clinical experience with 252 aneurysms in 168 patients. *Ann Surg.* 2001;234(4):454–462.
2. Chung R, Touska P, Morgan R, Belli AM. Endovascular management of true renal arterial aneurysms: Results from a single centre. *Cardiovasc Intervent Radiol.* 2016;39(1):36–43.
3. Chaer RA, Abularrage CJ, Coleman DM, et al. The Society for Vascular Surgery clinical practice guidelines on the management of visceral aneurysm. *J Vasc Surg.* 2020;72(1S):3S–39S.

30

Open and Laparoscopic Treatment of Median Arcuate Ligament Syndrome

Few disease processes have raised controversy within the field of vascular surgery more than median arcuate ligament syndrome.

JIMENEZ ET AL.

Research Question: What is the evidence for open and laparoscopic treatment in patients with median arcuate ligament syndrome (MALS)?[1]

Funding: None

Year Range for Searches: 1963–2012

Year Study Published: 2012

Number of Studies Included in Systematic Review: 20 studies

Which Studies Were Included: To be eligible for inclusion, studies had to present original data on the surgical management of MALS. Studies could be either retrospective or prospective.

Which Studies Were Excluded: Case series containing fewer than three patients and individual case reports were excluded. Patients within reported series were excluded if they did not undergo surgical intervention.

Patients: 400

Study Overview: A systematic review was conducted to identify the available literature on the clinical effectiveness of open and laparoscopic treatment for MALS. A comprehensive search strategy of the English literature was used with the following terms: celiac artery compression, celiac band compression, MAL compression, and Dunbar's syndrome.

Follow-up: Follow-up ranged from 10 to 229 months in the open group and from 6 to 44 months in the laparoscopic group.

Endpoints: The outcome measures were clinical improvement and intraoperative and postoperative complications.

RESULTS

- 20 suitable studies including 400 patients were identified for the review, with 13 investigating open MAL division and seven laparoscopic MAL division.
- All patients underwent either laparoscopic (n = 121) or open (n = 279) MAL division. 70 patients (25%) in the open series underwent concomitant arterial reconstruction. 11 patients (9%) underwent celiac artery angioplasty and stenting following laparoscopic MAL release.
- The most common presenting signs and symptoms for patients undergoing both treatment modalities were abdominal pain (80%), weight loss (48%) abdominal bruit (35%), nausea (9.7%), and diarrhea (7.5%).
- 339 patients (85%) reported immediate postoperative symptom relief, which included 218 out of 279 patients in the open group (78%) and 116 out of 121 in the laparoscopic group (96%). Late recurrence of symptoms was reported in 19 patients in the open group (6.8%) and seven patients in the laparoscopic group (5.7%).
- 11 out of 121 patients (9.1%) in the laparoscopic group required open conversion secondary to bleeding. Intraoperative complications in the laparoscopic group included visceral artery bleeding (4.1%), pneumothorax (2.5%), aortic bleeding (1.7%), and phrenic artery laceration (0.8%). Postoperative complications reported following laparoscopic repair included pancreatitis (0.8%) and gastroparesis (0.8%). No procedure-related deaths were reported in any of the laparoscopic series.
- In the open group, the incidence of major postoperative complications was 6.5%. The most common reported complication was thrombosis of a bypass graft (2%). Additional complications following open repair were

stroke (1.4%), gastroesophageal reflux disease (1%), pancreatitis (1%), hemothorax (0.3%), and splenic infarction (0.3%). No procedure-related deaths were reported in any of the open series.

Criticisms and Limitations: Because this was an observational study, it is not possible to rigorously compare the relative benefits and risks of different management strategies.

Due to the relatively short-term follow-up of patients treated by either laparoscopic MAL division with or without celiac stenting, or open division with or without arterial reconstruction, no conclusions could be drawn with respect to the durability of the various approaches.

It should also be noted that a limitation of summarizing data from small individual series may lead to publication bias toward success, magnifying the apparent benefit of the procedure.

Other Relevant Studies and Information

- An analysis involving 100 patients suffering from MALS showed that operative management of MALS can be performed with a low rate of complications. It also concluded that approximately two-thirds of questionnaire respondents were free of symptoms 5 years after the procedure.[2]
- A new treatment option for MALS is robotic-assisted release, and a case series of 13 patients treated with this method concluded that it was safe and efficacious in selected patients.[3]

Summary and Implications: For patients with MALS, this analysis demonstrated that both laparoscopic and open MAL release with celiac artery revascularization (open and endovascular) may provide sustained symptom relief in the majority of symptomatic patients.

CLINICAL CASE: MALS

Case History

A 51-year-old female patient is referred to your clinic by one of your gastroenterology colleagues. She has a 1-year history of intermittent epigastric pain worsened by eating, nausea, and weight loss. Thus far, the results of all investigations (esophagogastroduodenoscopy [OGD], colonoscopy, and barium swallow) have been normal, apart from a computed tomography scan showing a celiac artery stenosis and possible extrinsic compression by the MAL. How would you manage this patient?

Suggested Answer

The patient should undergo an ultrasound duplex by an experienced operator to confirm the celiac artery stenosis and to detect changes in peak systolic velocity during maximal inspiration and expiration. The findings are consistent with MALS, and following a multidisciplinary team meeting, the patient is counseled on the potential benefits of laparoscopic MAL release and its complications, which she accepts. She makes an uneventful recovery with complete relief from her symptoms, which is maintained with weight gain at 6 weeks of follow-up.

References

1. Jimenez JC, Harlander-Locke M, Dutson EP. Open and laparoscopic treatment of median arcuate ligament syndrome. *J Vasc Surg.* 2012;56(3):869–873.
2. Pather K, Kärkkäinen JM, Tenorio ER, et al. Long-term symptom improvement and health-related quality of life after operative management of median arcuate ligament syndrome. *J Vasc Surg.* 2021;73(6):2050–2058.
3. Khrucharoen U, Juo YY, Sanaiha Y, et al. Robotic-assisted laparoscopic median arcuate ligament release: 7-year experience from a single tertiary care center. *Surg Endosc.* 2018;32(9):4029–4035.

Peripheral Arterial Disease

JULIEN AL SHAKARCHI AND LEWIS MEECHAM

31

Supervised Exercise Versus Primary Stenting for Claudication Resulting from Aortoiliac Peripheral Artery Disease

The Claudication: Exercise Versus Endoluminal Revascularization (CLEVER) Study

This study demonstrates that for patients with claudication, supervised exercise provides a superior improvement in treadmill walking performance compared to both primary aortoiliac stent revascularization and optimal medical care.

THE CLEVER INVESTIGATORS

Research Question: What is the optimal treatment strategy for patients with claudication due to aortoiliac peripheral artery disease?[1]

Funding: The National Heart, Lung and Blood Institute, part of the National Institutes of Health

Year Study Began: 2007

Year Study Published: 2011

Study Location: 22 clinical centers from Canada and the US

Who Was Studied: Patients with symptoms of moderate to severe intermittent claudication (defined as ability to walk at least 2 but not more than 11 minutes on a graded treadmill) and objective evidence of a hemodynamically significant aortoiliac arterial stenosis.

Who Was Excluded: Individuals with critical limb ischemia or those who had comorbid conditions that limited their walking ability were excluded.

Patients: 111

Study Overview

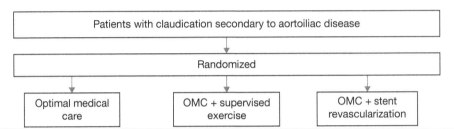

Figure 31.1 Design of CLEVER randomized controlled trial

Study Intervention: Patients were randomly assigned to receive one of three treatments: optimal medical care (OMC), OMC + supervised exercise, or OMC + stent revascularization. OMC consisted of risk-factor management, including antiplatelet use and home exercise and diet advice. All study participants also received cilostazol (100 mg twice daily). Supervised exercise consisted of 26 weeks of exercise, three times a week, for 1 hour at a time. Stent revascularization was carried out to relieve all hemodynamically significant stenoses (50% by diameter) in the aorta and iliac arteries.

Follow-up: 6 months

Endpoints: *Primary outcome measure:* Change from baseline to 6 months in the peak walking time on a graded treadmill test (Gardner protocol). *Secondary outcome measures:* Changes in the following parameters: claudication onset time, change in community-based walking as assessed by pedometer measurements over 7 consecutive days, self-reported walking and quality of life (QOL), and biomarkers of cardiovascular disease risk.

RESULTS

- 61% of study participants were men and the mean age was 64. Of those enrolled, 50% were current smokers and 23% were undergoing treatment for diabetes mellitus. <5% had had a previous endovascular intervention and 15% were taking cilostazol.
- In the revascularization group, ~70% required treatment of the common iliac artery; the rest underwent treatment of the external iliac artery, and one patient underwent aortic stenting. 38% of those treated had total occlusions; mean lesion length was 3.9 cm and mean degree of stenosis was 80% (Table 31.1).

Table 31.1 OUTCOME MEASURES IN THE THREE GROUPS

	OMC	OMC + supervised exercise	OMC + stent revascularization
Improvement in peak walking time (min)	1.2 ± 2.6	**5.8 ± 4.6** **(p = 0.001)**	3.7 ± 4.9 (p = 0.019)
Change in claudication onset time (min)	0.7 ± 1.1	3.0 ± 2.9 (p = 0.003)	**3.6 ± 4.2** **(p = 0.006)**
Change in ABPI (mmHg)	0.01 ± 0.10	0.03 ± 0.11 (p = 0.578)	**0.29 ± 0.33** **(p = 0.001)**

p values in boxes are results compared to control (OMC group).

- All groups demonstrated an increase in community-based walking; however, there was no difference among the three groups (suggesting this element is limited by lifestyle rather than disease).
- All groups showed QOL improvement; no significant difference was seen among the groups in either disease-related or generic QOL. On further analysis those patients with the best improvement in peak walking time had the highest improvement in QOL scores.
- Of note, there were four adverse events in the intervention group (compared to zero in the OMC and supervised exercise groups): One patient required transfusion, one had thrombosis requiring further stenting, and two had dissections of the iliac arteries.

Criticisms and Limitations: The follow-up period of this analysis was just 6 months, limiting the ability to draw conclusions about long-term outcomes.

No data on cost of care were provided, limiting the ability to draw conclusions about the relative cost-effectiveness of each approach.

Finally, a major factor that could have confounded results was concurrent femoropopliteal disease. Those patients with concurrent femoropopliteal disease may not have improved as significantly as those who did not have such disease. A breakdown of infra-inguinal disease should have been provided for all groups.

Other Relevant Studies and Information

- The Invasive Revascularization or Not in Intermittent Claudication (IRONIC) study (see Chapter 32)[2] came to similar conclusions as this analysis that there is no benefit to routine revascularization of patients with intermittent claudication as well as optimal medical therapy and regular exercise. This was also the conclusion of a Cochrane review on the topic.[3]
- Indeed, there are some data (real-world case series, with some methodological flaws) suggesting that intervention for intermittent claudication may in fact increase the likelihood of progression into chronic limb-threatening ischemia.[4]
- The 2016 American Heart Association/American College of Cardiology guidelines on the management of patients with lower-extremity peripheral artery disease recommend that patients with claudication should be offered a supervised exercise program to improve functional status and QOL and to reduce leg symptoms.[5]

Summary and Implications: In this trial of patients with intermittent claudication and aortoiliac arterial stenosis, supervised exercise and stent revascularization provided significant benefits with respect to peak walking time relative to optimal medical treatment alone; however, supervised exercise proved at least as effective as revascularization. This trial supports the optimization of medical treatment for patient with intermittent claudication as well as enrollment in a supervised exercise program, with stent revascularization reserved for those patients who fail to improve with the first two interventions.

CLINICAL CASE: AORTOILIAC DISEASE CAUSING INTERMITTENT CLAUDICATION

Case History

A 62-year-old man is referred to the vascular clinic with intermittent claudication in the calf and thigh of the left leg. This has been persisting for 6 months and has progressively worsened to the point he is now avoiding exercise. He reports being able to walk for only 3 minutes before having to rest. He is a current smoker, is a medicated hypertensive and non–insulin-dependent diabetic, and is not taking an antiplatelet medication. He is a retired schoolteacher and has a BMI of 36. On examination he has a full complement of pulses in the right leg and no palpable pulses in the left leg. Ankle–brachial pressure index (ABPI) was 0.68. A treadmill test was performed; the patient terminated the test at 2 minutes 26 seconds with no incline. Duplex ultrasonography revealed >90% stenosis of the left common iliac artery.

Suggested Answer

This patient is suffering from moderate to severe intermittent claudication secondary to a tight left common iliac artery stenosis. His medical treatment is not optimal: He should be offered smoking cessation and started on an antiplatelet (ideally clopidogrel 75 mg) and high-intensity statin therapy (atorvastatin 80 mg). He should be enrolled in a supervised exercise program and encouraged to attend. He should be reviewed in 6 months to assess his progress. If his walking distance has not improved and he has been compliant with OMT, then revascularization should be considered.

References

1. Murphy TP, Cutlip DE, Regensteiner JG, et al. Supervised exercise versus primary stenting for claudication resulting from aortoiliac peripheral artery disease. *Circulation*. 2012;125(1):130–139. doi:10.1161/CIRCULATIONAHA.111.075770
2. Djerf H, Millinger J, Falkenberg M, et al. Absence of long-term benefit of revascularization in patients with intermittent claudication: Five-year results from the IRONIC randomized controlled trial. *Circ Cardiovasc Interv*. 2020;13:e008450. DOI:10.1161/CIRCINTERVENTIONS.119.008450
3. Jansen SC, Abaraogu UO, Lauret GJ, et al. Modes for exercise training for intermittent claudication. *Cochrane Database Syst Rev*. 2020;8(8):CD009638. DOI:10.1002/14651858.CD009638.pub3
4. Madabhushi V, Davenport D, Jones S, et al. Revascularization of intermittent claudicants leads to more chronic limb-threatening ischaemia and higher amputation rates. *J Vasc Surg*. 2021;74(3):771–779. DOI:10.1016/j/jvs.2021.02.045
5. Gerhard-Herman MD, Gornik HL, Barrett C, et al. 2016 AHA/ACC guideline on the management of patients with lower extremity peripheral artery disease: A report of the American College of Cardiology/American Heart Association Task Force on Clinical Practice Guidelines. *Circulation*. 2017;135(12):e726–e779.

32

Absence of Long-Term Benefit of Revascularization in Patients with Intermittent Claudication

The Invasive Revascularization or Not in Intermittent Claudication (IRONIC) Study

> Revascularization was not found to be a cost-effective option.
> THE IRONIC INVESTIGATORS

Research Question: What is the long-term effectiveness and cost-effectiveness of revascularization compared with a noninvasive approach for intermittent claudication (IC)?[1]

Funding: The Fred G. and Emma E. Kanold Foundation, the Gothenburg Medical Society, the Helena Althin Foundation, the Swedish Heart and Lung Foundation, the Hjalmar Svensson Foundation, the Swedish Research Council, and grants from the Swedish state under the agreement between the Swedish government and the county councils

Year Study Began: 2010

Year Study Published: 2020

Study Location: One clinical center in Sweden

Who Was Studied: Patients <80 years of age with a confirmed diagnosis of unilateral or bilateral lifestyle-limiting mild to severe IC (lasting >6 months) and with corresponding atherosclerotic lesions in the aortoiliac and femoropopliteal segment, as verified by duplex ultrasound, were eligible for the trial.

Who Was Excluded: Exclusion criteria were severe claudication prohibiting basic everyday activities, critical limb ischemia, mild nonlimiting symptoms, two or more previously failed ipsilateral invasive procedures, and failure to complete the Swedish versions of health-related quality-of-life (HRQoL) assessments.

Patients: 158

Study Overview

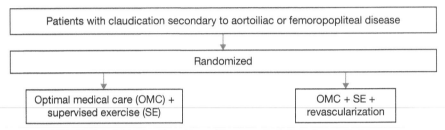

Figure 32.1 Design of IRONIC randomized controlled trial

Study Intervention: Patients were randomly assigned to revascularization in addition to best medical treatment and exercise therapy (the revascularization group) or best medical treatment and exercise therapy alone (the nonrevascularization group).

Follow-up: Mean follow-up of 5.2 years

Endpoints: *Primary outcome measure:* HRQoL change assessed with the generic medical outcomes study short form 36 (SF-36). *Secondary outcome measures:* HRQoL change assessed with the vascular quality-of-life questionnaire, IC distance, and maximum walking distance.

RESULTS

- 77.5% of eligible patients were enrolled into the trial. 73% of those completed 5-year follow-up (84% of those who were alive).
- Mean age was 68 years, 30% of the cohort were current smokers, 20% had diabetes mellitus, and BMI was ~25.

- Of the 79 patients randomized to revascularization, 70 (90%) underwent a revascularization procedure. 28/70 (40%) underwent intervention for aortoiliac disease and 45/70 (64%) had a femoropopliteal intervention; some (not specified) had a combination of aortoiliac and femoropopliteal treatments. 22 (28%) underwent a secondary intervention during the study period.
- Both groups showed improvement in terms of the physical component of the SF-36 questionnaire (p ≤ 0.05). Both groups demonstrated improvement in terms of IC distance at 5 years (non-revascularization, +55 m; revascularization, +51 m, p = 0.001). However, there was no improvement in maximal walking distance (non-revascularization, +14 m; revascularization, –12 m). Ankle–brachial pressure index (APBI) was higher in the revascularization group compared to the non-revascularization group (0.83 vs. 0.76, p = 0.04).
- In terms of cost-effectiveness, invasive treatment was estimated to be $5,849–$6,133 more expensive during the study period. There were a similar number of quality-adjusted life-years (QALYs) gained by both groups (non-revascularization 3.04 vs. revascularization 2.88), making invasive treatment not cost-effective compared to noninvasive treatment for IC. On multiple imputation analysis, cost per QALY for invasive treatment was $5.5 million.

Criticisms and Limitations: The methodology of this trial is robust and clear; it provides an answer to the question it was designed to investigate. There are, however, some limitations. As a single-center study, there will be a question as to the generalizability of the findings and whether the types of intervention performed introduce systematic bias due to the treatment habits of the investigating center.

Second, the definition of supervised exercise is not as comprehensive as it is in other studies. In this study patients were given written and verbal information on exercise for 30 minutes 3 days a week and were seen at 3 and 6 months; no other supervision was provided. One would argue that these goals for exercise are far below what would be considered adequate exercise levels for improving IC.[2]

Finally, the heterogeneity of the pattern of disease may have confounded the results. It may be that those with aortoiliac disease improved more than those with combined aortoiliac and femoropopliteal disease as a result of surgical treatment.

Other Relevant Studies and Information

- The results of this study echo those of the Claudication: Exercise Versus Endoluminal Revascularization (CLEVER)[3] study published in 2012, which also found no benefit of revascularization over optimal medical therapy and exercise (see Chapter 31).
- A Cochrane review in 2018 found 10 randomized controlled trials for comparison. They concluded there was no additional benefit of revascularization in terms of walking distance and HRQoL over optimal medical therapy and exercise.[4]
- A more recent meta-analysis concluded the same, indicating that even home-based exercise may provide equivalent results.[5]
- The 2016 American Heart Association/American College of Cardiology guidelines on the management of patients with lower-extremity peripheral artery disease recommend that patients with claudication should be offered a supervised exercise program to improve functional status and quality of life and to reduce leg symptoms.[6]

Summary and Implications: This trial of patients with IC due to vascular disease failed to demonstrate a benefit of surgical revascularization in addition to optimal medical management and supervised exercise for improving quality of life. The study also highlighted that surgical revascularization is not cost-effective, with an additional cost of $5.5 million to achieve 1 QALY. These findings are consistent with other research on the topic.

CLINICAL CASE: IC AND INFRA-INGUINAL DISEASE

Case History

A 68-year-old female who is an ex-smoker and suffers from hypertension attends the vascular clinic with IC of >6 months' duration. She reports being able to walk for 5 minutes on the flat before having to stop due to pain in the right calf. There are also symptoms on the left, but they are less severe. Apart from treatment for hypertension she is not taking any other medicines. She is retired but is sociable and desperate to travel more with her group of friends but finds that having to stop walking is slowing her and the group down. On examination there are femoral pulses bilaterally; on the left she has weak popliteal and pedal pulses and on the right there are no pulses below the femoral artery. ABPI on the right side is 0.8. How should this patient be treated?

Suggested Answer

She should be established on best medical therapy in terms of antiplatelet therapy (clopidogrel 75 mg OD) and high-intensity statin therapy (atorvastatin 80 mg ON). Her blood pressure should be controlled adequately. It is likely she has significant superficial femoral or popliteal disease on the right. Investigation in terms of duplex ultrasonography may be performed, but regardless of the results the treatment (in the initial phase) should remain the same. She should be enrolled in the local supervised exercise program and monitored clinically for 6 months.

References

1. Djerf H, Millinger J, Falkenberg M, et al. Absence of long-term benefit of revascularization in patients with intermittent claudication: Five-year results from the IRONIC randomized controlled trial. *Circ Cardiovasc Interv.* 2020;13:e008450. DOI:10.1161/CIRCINTERVENTIONS.119.008450
2. Jansen SC, Abaraogu UO, Lauret GJ, et al. Modes for exercise training for intermittent claudication. *Cochrane Databse Syst Rev.* 2020;8(8):CD009638. DOI:10.1002/14651858.CD009638.pub3
3. Murphy TP, Cutlip DE, Regensteiner JG, et al. Supervised exercise versus primary stenting for claudication resulting from aortoiliac peripheral artery disease. *Circulation.* 2012;125(1):130–139. DOI:10.1161/CIRCULATIONAHA.111.075770
4. Fakhry F, Fokkenrood HJP, Spronk S, et al. Endovascular revascularisation of intermittent claudication (pain in the legs). *Cochrane Database Syst Rev.* 2018;2018(3):CD010512.
5. Van den Houten MML, Hageman D, Gommans LNM, et al. The effect of supervised exercise, home-based exercise and endovascular revascularisation on physical activity in patients with intermittent claudication: A network meta-analysis. *Eur J Vasc Endovasc Surg.* 2019;58(3):383–392. DOI:10.1016/j.ejvs.2018.12.023
6. Gerhard-Herman MD, Gornik HL, Barrett C, et al. 2016 AHA/ACC guidelines on the management of patients with lower extremity peripheral artery disease: A report of the American College of Cardiology/American Heart Association Task Force on Clinical Practice Guidelines. *Circulation.* 2017;135(12):e726–e779.

33

Autologous Saphenous Vein and Expanded Polytetrafluoroethylene Grafts in Infra-inguinal Arterial Reconstructions

A 6-Year Prospective Multicenter Randomized Comparison

> Femoropopliteal bypasses performed with randomized [polytetrafluoro-ethylene] grafts have patency rates inferior to those performed with randomized [autologous saphenous vein] grafts.
>
> VEITH ET AL.

Research Question: Is there any difference in outcome between autologous saphenous vein (ASV) grafts and expanded polytetrafluoroethylene (PTFE) grafts in infra-inguinal arterial reconstructions?[1]

Funding: Manning, Brown, and Seabury Foundations

Year Study Began: 1978

Year Study Published: 1986

Study Location: Three clinical centers in the US

Who Was Studied: Patients were eligible if they required a bypass to the popliteal or an infra-popliteal artery to control ischemia caused by arteriosclerosis.

Who Was Excluded: Patients with infra-inguinal arteriosclerosis who could be treated solely by a deep femoral artery reconstruction or solely by percutaneous angioplasty were excluded from the study.

Patients: 759 patients were enrolled and underwent 845 bypass procedures.

Study Overview

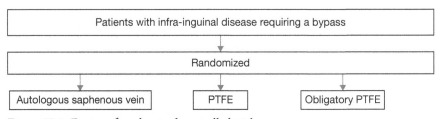

Figure 33.1 Design of randomized controlled trial

Study Intervention: Patients were randomly assigned to either ASV or PTFE bypass if they were suitable for both. If there was no autologous vein option, obligatory PTFE was chosen.

Follow-up: Up to 5 years

Endpoints: The main outcome measures were graft patency and limb salvage.

RESULTS

- Distribution of randomization to groups was relatively even. There were equivalent rates of gangrene/ulcer/tissue loss/claudication and diabetes mellitus among all six groups. A relatively high number of these patients were diagnosed with diabetes (62%). ~90% of the interventions were for patients suffering from chronic limb-threatening ischemia (CLTI). Mean age of the cohort was 70 years, with no mention of sex distribution.
- ASV and randomized PTFE bypass to the popliteal arteries had equivalent patency out to 2 years, at which point the performance of PTFE significantly declined. For the whole cohort, the 5-year patency was 68% versus 38% (p = 0.025) for ASV and PTFE respectively.
- When analyzed by distal anastomosis to the above-the-knee or below-the-knee popliteal artery, there was a nonsignificant trend toward worse patency rates with PTFE in the above-the-knee group (61% vs. 38%,

p > 0.25); in the below-the-knee group, patency rates with PTFE were significantly worse (76% vs. 54%, p < 0.05).

- Interestingly, in those patients deemed to have better runoff (popliteal artery running into ≥5 cm of tibial vessel), patency rates were improved in both groups but were still significantly better in the ASV bypass group (at 4 years 73% vs. 54%, p = 0.025).
- Despite the superior patency of ASV bypass grafts, there was no significant difference in rates of limb salvage between the two groups at 5 years (75% vs. 70%, p = 0.25).
- In terms of primary patency in the infra-popliteal segment, ASV bypass outperformed PTFE bypass for the whole study period (at 5 years 49% vs. 12%, p < 0.001). Again, this did not translate into improved limb salvage (57% vs. 61%, p = 0.5).
- Primary patency for obligatory PTFE bypass was inferior in both femoropopliteal cohorts and infra-popliteal cohorts. At 5 years, obligatory PTFE had significantly worse primary patency compared to those randomized to PTFE bypass in the femoropopliteal cohort (47% vs. 29%, p < 0.025) but not in the infra-popliteal cohort (12% vs. 7%, p > 0.5). Despite the poor patency rates, out to 4 years, limb salvage was equivalent in the femoropopliteal group (69% vs. 68%, p = 0.25) but significantly worse in the infra-popliteal group (61% vs. 19%, p = 0.01).

Criticisms and Limitations

- This randomized study was conducted prior to the era of electronic data capture and sophisticated statistical analysis packages. There are factors to consider when interpreting the data. For instance, we do not have a full picture of the comorbid nature of the patients; there could have been significant differences between the groups at baseline.
- There is a lack of information on best medical therapy and active smoking in the cohort of patients, which can have a direct impact on graft patency. Although the authors attempted to standardize preoperative and postoperative antiplatelet use, they acknowledge that this was not uniform across the participating centers and cannot guarantee patient compliance once discharged.
- In addition, there is no detail on the survival rates in the groups and how this affected analysis. Secondary procedures for limb salvage was not described and might have been a factor in limb-salvage rates if patients had a subsequent vein bypass following a failed PTFE graft.

Other Relevant Studies and Information
- A Cochrane review published in 2018 analyzed the optimal conduit for lower-limb bypass surgery. 19 randomized controlled trials were included for analysis (3,123 patients). The majority of the patients underwent above-the-knee popliteal bypass (n = 2,547). The authors concluded that vein bypass was the conduit of choice, and that non-reinforced Dacron has superior primary patency compared to PTFE. The use of a Miller cuff in conjunction with a synthetic conduit did not confer any benefit in terms of patency. Lack of data for below-the-knee bypass and poorly reported limb-salvage rates prevented conclusions from being drawn on these key issues.[2]
- Both UK National Institute for Health and Care Excellence (NICE) guidelines and the global vascular clinical guidelines recommend the use of percutaneous angioplasty before the use of a synthetic conduit for bypass for revascularization of patients with CLTI.[3,4]

Summary and Implications: In this trial of patients requiring bypass surgery for peripheral arterial disease, patients who received ASV grafting had higher patency rates than those treated with PTFE. Nevertheless, there were no significant differences in limb-salvage rates between the groups. Still, because of the superior patency rates, vein grafting is the preferred option if it is feasible, with PTFE reserved for patients with no suitable venous conduit.

CLINICAL CASE: CHOICE OF CONDUIT FOR INFRA-INGUINAL BYPASS

Case History
A 70-year-old female has been admitted via the emergency department with hallux gangrene of the right leg and pain at rest in the foot. She is an ex-smoker, has a history of ischemic heart disease (myocardial infarction 4 years ago), and is a type 2 diabetic taking insulin. She is taking clopidogrel and high-intensity statin as well as bisoprolol and ramipril. Examination confirms she is suffering from CLTI: She has femoral pulses only in both lower limbs and her ankle–brachial pressure index (ABPI) is 0.18. Computed tomographic (CT) angiography confirms a full-length occlusion of the superficial femoral artery and stenotic disease of her above-the-knee popliteal artery. She has a patent below-the-knee popliteal artery with two-vessel runoff via the posterior tibial and

peroneal arteries. Vein map reveals borderline great saphenous vein (GSV) in both legs (~3–3.5 mm). Which treatment would you offer this patient?

Suggested Answer

Revascularization is mandated in patients with CLTI who are fit for intervention. Given the length of her disease (Global Limb Anatomic Staging System [GLASS] stage 3), surgical bypass would be the most appropriate option. The gold standard would be vein bypass with the ipsilateral GSV. Preoperative ultrasound scan reveals that this woman has borderline GSV in both legs. It may be that these veins are appropriate for use, or maybe on surgical exploration it is found that they are not sufficient for use as a conduit. At that point, if that is the case intraoperatively, the patient should undergo synthetic bypass as the limb-salvage rates are comparable.

References

1. Veith FJ, Gupta SK, Ascer E, et al. Six-year prospective multicenter randomized comparison of autologous saphenous vein and expanded polytetrafluoroethylene grafts in infrainguinal arterial reconstructions. *J Vasc Surg.* 1996;3(1):104–114.
2. Ambler GK, Twine CP. Graft type for femoro-popliteal bypass surgery. *Cochrane Database Syst Rev.* 2018;2(2):CD001487.
3. National Institute for Health and Care Excellence (NICE). Peripheral arterial disease: Diagnosis and management. 2020. https://www.nice.org.uk/guidance/cg147
4. Conte MS, Bradbury AW, Kolh P, et al. Global vascular guidelines on the management of chronic limb-threatening ischemia. *J Vasc Surg.* 2019;69:3S–125S.

34

Bypass Versus Angioplasty in Severe Ischemia of the Leg (BASIL)

A Multicenter, Randomized Controlled Trial

> Severe limb ischemia imposes a very high human cost as well as a major economic burden on health and social care.
>
> THE BASIL INVESTIGATORS

Research Question: What are the outcomes of a surgery-first strategy and an angioplasty-first strategy in patients with severe limb ischemia?

Funding: UK National Health Service (NHS) and Research and Development Health Technology Assessment (HTA) Programme

Year Study Began: 1999

Year Study Published: 2005

Study Location: 27 clinical centers in the UK

Who Was Studied: Patients were included if they presented with severe limb ischemia, defined as rest pain or tissue loss (ulcer or gangrene) of presumed arterial etiology for >2 weeks, and who on diagnostic imaging had a pattern of disease that could be treated by either infra-inguinal bypass surgery or balloon angioplasty.

Who Was Excluded: No exclusion criteria specifically mentioned in the text

Patients: 452

Study Overview

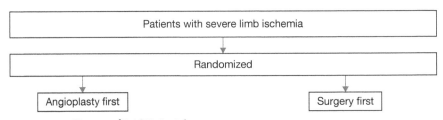

Figure 34.1 Design of BASIL 1 trial

Study Intervention: Patients were randomly assigned to receive either surgery first or angioplasty first.

Follow-up: 442 (99%) patients had been followed up at 1 year, 336 (74%) at 2 years, 216 (48%) at 3 years, 99 (22%) at 4 years, and 37 (8%) at 5 years.

Endpoints: *Primary outcome measure:* Time to amputation of the trial leg above the ankle or death from any cause, whichever occurred first (i.e., amputation-free survival [AFS]). *Secondary outcomes:* All-cause mortality, 30-day morbidity and mortality, reinterventions, health-related quality of life (HRQoL), and use of hospital resources.

RESULTS

- Baseline demographic data were similar in the two groups, confirming an appropriate randomization strategy. Two thirds of the cohort were age >70 years. 60% of participants were male, 40% had diabetes mellitus, 30% had bilateral symptomatic peripheral arterial disease, and 75% had tissue loss on the foot.
- Best medical therapy rates were low: statin therapy ~33%, antiplatelet therapy ~55%, antihypertensive treatment ~60%, and ~33% were current smokers. Only eight patients were lost to follow-up at the end of the trial.
- There was no significant difference in AFS between the two groups at 1 and 3 years (Table 34.1). There was no difference in rates of major lower-limb amputation between the two groups. Limb salvage at 12 months was ~80%. Patients randomized to receive surgery first had significantly fewer

reinterventions in the trial period (18% vs. 26%, AR 8%, 95% confidence interval 4–15%).

- A post-hoc analysis, done after examination of the survival curves, showed a significantly reduced hazard in AFS (adjusted hazard ratio [HR] 0.37 [95% CI 0.17–0.77], p = 0.008) and all-cause mortality (0.34 [0.17–0.71], p = 0.004) for surgery relative to angioplasty in the period beyond 2 years from randomization.

Table 34.1 AFS AT 1 AND 3 YEARS SHOWING NO SIGNIFICANT DIFFERENCE

	Surgery first	Angioplasty first
AFS at 1 year	68%	71%
AFS at 3 years	57%	52%

- HRQoL (measured with EQ5D and SF36) improved in the first 3 months (no difference between treatment arms) and then remained static.
- The mean cost of inpatient hospital treatment during the first 12 months of follow-up in patients assigned to a surgery-first strategy was estimated as £23,322 (£20,096 hospital stay, £3,225 procedure costs), which is about a third higher than the £17,419 (£15,381, £2,039) for patients assigned an angioplasty-first strategy.

Criticisms and Limitations: The trial took longer than anticipated to recruit its target population, and ~61% of patients were recruited from only six centers. Also, the BASIL audit revealed that only 20% of eligible patients were recruited into the trial. These factors have led to questioning the generalizability of the trial. Also, 75% of patients underwent femoropopliteal intervention, and thus the findings may not be applicable to patients with other types of peripheral vascular disease.

Other Relevant Studies and Information

- The BASIL trial is still the only randomized controlled trial to compare an angioplasty-first versus a surgery-first approach for infra-inguinal revascularization of patients with chronic limb-threatening ischemia (CLTI). However, other small and less rigorous analyses show similar findings.[4,5]
- A similar trial was attempted in the Netherlands for patients with symptomatic superficial femoral artery occlusions (5–15 cm)[2]. 56 patients were recruited to either bypass or angioplasty, with bypass having far superior primary patency at 12 months (three bypasses

required to avoid one occlusion). Others have tried to conduct similar trials and not been able to gather enough data for publication.[3]
• The Global Vascular Guidelines[6] recommend using endovascular revascularization for patients who are at high surgical risk, have relatively simple disease, or have low to moderate foot threat.

Summary and Implications: The BASIL trial showed that for patients with severe limb ischemia due to peripheral arterial disease, angioplasty and surgical revascularization result in similar AFS rates. In a post-hoc analysis, patients undergoing open surgery had modestly better outcomes beyond 2 years. Based on this and other research, the Global Vascular Guidelines recommend endovascular revascularization for patients who have relatively simple disease or who are at high surgical risk.

CLINICAL CASE: ENDOVASCULAR OR OPEN THERAPY FOR SUPERFICIAL FEMORAL ARTERY DISEASE

Case History
A 62-year-old man presents to the vascular clinic with a long history of intermittent claudication, but over the last 2 weeks he has developed gangrene of the right hallux. He is an ex-smoker and suffers from type 2 diabetes mellitus, hypertension, and degenerative lumbar disease. Currently he is taking metformin and ramipril with co-codamol (a mixture of acetaminophen and codeine) as needed. His BMI is 38. He has good femoral pulses bilaterally with nothing palpable below. There are audible monophasic posterior tibial (PT) and dorsalis pedis (DP) signals with an ankle–brachial pressure index (ABPI) of 0.34. Duplex ultrasonography reveals full-length occlusion of the superficial femoral artery with some calcified disease of the above-the-knee popliteal artery; otherwise, he has patent runoff from the below-the-knee popliteal artery. The great saphenous vein (GSV) is 4 mm wide throughout its length.

Suggested Answer
This patient has standard comorbidities for a patient with CLTI. As he has an adequate GSV and a low comorbidity burden (likely to survive >2 years), the options should be discussed with the patient and it should be explained to him that he is likely to benefit more in the long term from an open surgical bypass.

References

1. The BASIL Trial Participants. Bypass versus angioplasty in severe ischaemia of the leg (BASIL): Multicentre, randomised controlled trial. *Lancet.* 2005;366:1925–1934. DOI:10.1016/S0140-6736(05)67704-5

2. Van der Zaag ES, Legemate DA, Prins MH, et al. Angioplasty or bypass for superficial artery disease? A randomised controlled trial. *Eur J Vasc Endovasc Surg.* 2004;28(2):132–137.

3. Malas MB, Qazi U, Glebova N, et al. Design of the revascularization with Open Bypass vs. Angioplasty and Stenting of the Lower Extremity Trial (ROBUST). *JAMA Surg.* 2014;149(12):1289–1295. DOI:10.1001/jamasurg.2014.369

4. Almasari J, Adusumalli J, Asi N, et al. Systematic review and meta-analysis of revascularization outcomes of infra-inguinal chronic limb-threatening ischaemia. *J Vasc Surg.* 2019;69(6):126S–136S. https://doi.org/10.1016/j.jvs.2018.01.071

5. Antoniou GA, Georgiadis GS, Antoniou SA, et al. Bypass surgery for chronic lower limb ischaemia. *Cochrane Database Syst Rev.* 2017;2017(4):CD002000.

6. Conte MS, Bradbury AW, Kolh P, et al. Global vascular guidelines on the management of chronic limb-threatening ischemia. *J Vasc Surg.* 2019;69:3S–125S.

35

Is Duplex Surveillance of Value After Leg Vein Bypass Grafting?

Principal Results of the Vein Graft Surveillance Randomized Trial (VGST)

This large [randomized controlled trial] has shown no clinical benefit or quality-of-life improvement in patients participating in a duplex surveillance program.

THE VGST INVESTIGATORS

Research Question: Is duplex surveillance of value following lower-limb vein bypass?

Funding: British Heart Foundation

Year Study Began: 1998

Year Study Published: 2005

Study Location: 29 clinical centers in the UK (22) and the rest of Europe (7)

Who Was Studied: Patients with peripheral arterial disease were eligible if they had undergone femoropopliteal or femorotibial bypasses and their vein graft was patent at 30 days after surgery.

Who Was Excluded: Patients receiving synthetic grafts (such as polytetrafluoro-ethylene [PTFE] or Dacron grafts) were excluded from the study.

Patients: 594

Study Overview

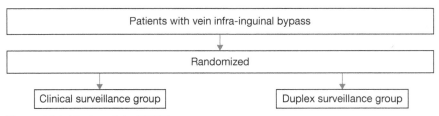

Figure 35.1 Design of the VGST

Study Intervention: Patients were randomly assigned to either the clinical group (clinical examination with ankle–brachial pressure index [ABPI] measurements) or the duplex group (same as the clinical group plus a routine duplex scan). Patients underwent a surveillance program with follow-up appointments at the time of recruitment (6 weeks) and then at 3, 6, 9, 12, and 18 months. The duplex group was scanned at every visit along the graft, including the distal and proximal anastomoses, while the clinical surveillance had a single scan at 18 months.

Follow-up: Mean follow-up of 5.2 years

Endpoints: *Primary outcomes:* Time to amputation and vascular mortality. *Secondary outcomes:* Patency, cost, and quality of life.

RESULTS

- Baseline demographic results were comparable for the two groups. The cohort had a median age of 70 years, 72% were male, and the median ABPI was 0.48. Clinical indications for the bypass were chronic limb-threatening ischemia (CLTI; two thirds of patients) and intermittent claudication (IC; one third of patients). In 92% of cases the ipsilateral great saphenous vein was used as the bypass conduit, and this was reversed in two thirds of the cases.
- Among enrolled patients, 12% withdrew from the trial (45% of these underwent major lower-limb amputation). 90% attended their clinical follow-up appointments and surveillance scan appointments; 90% had a

completion duplex scan at 18 months. Completion of quality-of-life data was slightly less, at 80%.

- Clinical interventions were more common in the duplex surveillance group (22% vs. 16%, p = 0.07), and time to intervention was earlier (15 weeks vs. 20 weeks). Reported technical success was 90% in both groups.

- Clinical outcomes, including amputation (7% vs. 7%), vascular death (3% vs. 4%), and amputation or vascular death (10% vs. 11%), were similar between the two groups. Radiologic outcomes were also similar for primary patency (69% vs. 67%), assisted primary patency (76% vs. 76%), and secondary patency (80% vs. 79%). There was no difference in health-related quality of life at 6 and 18 months (Table 35.1).

- Duplex surveillance, however, was associated with more cost than clinical surveillance, with a mean cost difference of £495 (95% confidence interval [CI] £183–£807, p = 0.002).

Table 35.1 MAJOR OUTCOMES IN THE CLINICAL AND DUPLEX FOLLOW-UP GROUPS

	Clinical surveillance (n = 290)	Duplex surveillance (n = 304)	Hazard ratio (95% CI)
Amputation	21 (7)	21 (7)	1.01 (0.55–1.86)
Vascular death	10 (3)	12 (4)	1.21 (0.52–2.81)
Amputation or vascular death	29 (10)	33 (11)	1.15 (0.70–1.90)
All deaths	31 (11)	36 (12)	1.22 (0.75–1.98)
Number of patients with 18 months of scanning	204	211	
Stenosis in graft at 18 months	39 (19)	25 (12)	

Criticisms and Limitations: Because this trial was limited to patients with a patent bypass without stenosis at 30 days, the findings may not be applicable to higher-risk patients.

Intensive clinical follow-up requires patients to be assessed (history, examination, and ABPI) frequently in the outpatient clinic. This intensive and frequent follow-up is not representative of the service that patients with CLTI normally receive and it may indicate that the control group performed better than they would in real-life settings. Therefore, it is important to highlight that the outcome of this trial is only applicable in settings with robust clinical surveillance.

Other Relevant Studies and Information

- This study was designed and funded as a consequence of two small studies by Lundell et al.[2] and Ihlberg et al.[3] that reported conflicting results with respect to the value of routine surveillance duplex studies after leg vein bypass grafting.
- A meta-analysis of 15 studies published in the *Journal of Vascular Surgery* in 2017[4] reported no difference in clinical outcomes or patency between the two surveillance options.
- UK National Institute for Health and Care Excellence (NICE) Clinical Guideline 147[5] does not make any comment on the appropriateness or methods of surveillance after lower-limb revascularization. The Global Vascular Guidelines[6] make a good practice statement (not based on evidence) that all patients undergoing lower-extremity bypass should be maintained in close clinical surveillance with the addition of ultrasound duplex where available.

Summary and Implications: This trial comparing clinical surveillance versus routine surveillance duplex studies after leg vein bypass grafting failed to demonstrate a benefit of routine duplex studies. In settings in which robust clinical follow-up is possible after leg vein bypass grafting, the addition of surveillance duplex scanning is unnecessary.

CLINICAL CASE: SURVEILLANCE FOLLOWING INFRA-INGUINAL BYPASS

Case History

A 70-year-old male with CLTI (gangrene of the second toe) has been assessed in the outpatient vascular clinic. He has a relatively low comorbidity burden (ex-smoker and hypertensive) and lives independently. His ABPI is 0.36 and he only has a palpable femoral pulse in the groin. Imaging of the arterial tree shows multilevel occlusive disease throughout the superficial femoral artery and popliteal artery. The case has been discussed by the multidisciplinary team and the consensus opinion was for a femoral tibioperoneal trunk (TPT) bypass with ipsilateral vein. You have performed this procedure without incident and the next day there is a posterior tibial (PT) pulse in the foot with an ABPI of 0.91. What will your follow-up arrangements be for this patient in terms of monitoring his vein bypass graft?

> **Suggested Answer**
> Patient can be enrolled in either clinical or duplex ultrasound surveillance, depending on the restrictions of the department. Clinical surveillance needs to be intensive, with clinical assessment and ABPI measurements at every visit.

References

1. Davies AH, Hawdon AJ, Sydes MR, Thompson SG. Is duplex surveillance of value after leg vein bypass grafting? Principal results of the Vein Graft Surveillance Randomised Trial (VGST). *Circulation*. 2005;112(13):1985–1991.
2. Lundell A, Lindblad B, Bergqvist D, Hansen F. Femoropopliteal-crural graft patency is improved by an intensive surveillance program: A prospective randomized study. *J Vasc Surg*. 1995;21:26–33.
3. Ihlberg L, Luther M, Tierala E, Lepantalo M. The utility of duplex scanning in infrainguinal vein graft surveillance: Results from a randomised controlled study. *Eur J Vasc Endovasc Surg*. 1998;16:19–27.
4. Abu Dabrh AM, Mohammed K, Farah W, et al. Systematic review and meta-analysis of duplex ultrasound surveillance for infrainguinal vein bypass grafts. *J Vasc Surg*. 2017;66(6):1885–1891.
5. National Institute for Health and Care Excellence (NICE). Peripheral arterial disease: Diagnosis and management. 2020. https://www.nice.org.uk/guidance/cg147
6. Conte MS, Bradbury AW, Kolh P, et al. Global vascular guidelines on the management of chronic limb-threatening ischemia. *J Vasc Surg*. 2019;69:3S–125S.

36

Dutch Iliac Stent Trial

Long-Term Results in Patients Randomized for Primary or Selective Stent Placement

Selective stent placement for iliac artery lesions results in a better preservation of symptomatic success in the long term.

THE DUTCH ILIAC STENT TRIAL INVESTIGATORS

Research Question: Does primary iliac stenting improve long-term outcomes compared with iliac angioplasty with selective stenting?[1]

Funding: Cordis

Year Study Began: 1993

Year Study Published: 2006

Study Location: Six clinical centers in the Netherlands

Who Was Studied: Inclusion criteria were:
- Clinical signs and symptoms of peripheral arterial disease (PAD) and/or reduced pulsation of the femoral artery and/or reduced ankle–brachial pressure index (ABPI)
- Significant stenosis in the common or external iliac artery—as evident by an arterial diameter reduction of >50% at angiography—and/or a peak systolic velocity ratio of >2.5 and/or a mean pressure gradient of >10 mmHg over the stenosis (with intra-arterial vasodilation)

- Stenosis of ≤10 cm in length or occlusion of ≤5 cm in length that allowed passage with a guidewire

Who Was Excluded: Patients were excluded if they were unwilling to participate, if the results of their angiography could not confirm the extent of disease as assessed with duplex ultrasonography, or if the patient had extensive aortoiliac disease or stenosis of >10 cm in length or occlusion of >5 cm.

Patients: 279

Study Overview

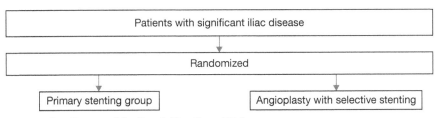

Figure 36.1 Design of the Dutch Iliac Stent Trial

Study Intervention: Patients were randomly assigned to either primary stent placement or primary percutaneous transluminal angioplasty (PTA) with selective stent placement in cases in which the residual mean pressure gradient was >10 mmHg across the treated site.

Follow-up: Mean follow-up of 6.3 years

Endpoints: The main outcome measures were symptomatic success (increase of at least one Fontaine grade during the whole follow-up period), hemodynamic success (increase of the ABPI of ≥0.10 during the whole follow-up period), iliac patency, and quality-of-life score.

RESULTS

- Median age was 58 years and ~60% of the cohort were men. 90% of the participants had Fontaine class II disease. Mean pre-intervention ABPI was 0.75.
- In terms of disease characteristics, the trial artery segment was the common iliac artery (CIA) in 70% of participants. The majority of the lesions were short stenosis (80% > 50% stenosis, 60% of lesions were

<2 cm in length); only 10% had chronic total occlusion of the arterial segment treated.

- 16–18% of the participants had a superficial femoral artery occlusion and 6–10% had profunda femoris artery occlusion.
- Stenting was performed in 97% of the primary stent group and 40% of the selective stenting group.
- At the final follow-up (6–8 years), 66% of the primary stent group and 51% of the selective stenting group had symptoms of peripheral arterial disease (hazard ratio [HR] = 0.8, 95% confidence interval [CI] 0.6–1.0).
- Patency was superior for the primary stent group (83% vs. 74%; HR = 1.3, 95% CI 0.8–2.1); however, there was no difference in terms of re-interventions (17% vs. 21%; HR = 1.1; 95% CI 0.6–1.9). No significant differences in quality of life were measured throughout the study period. No formal cost analysis was performed.

Criticisms and Limitations: It must be considered that the patients and lesions selected for the trial were relatively minor, and thus the findings might not apply to patients with more extensive disease.

It is noteworthy that despite worse patency, the angioplasty group had more symptomatic improvement. This is a common finding in arterial trials: Patency often doesn't translate into clinical benefit.

Other Relevant Studies and Information

- A 2020 Cochrane review[2] found that there was only one other trial investigating this topic for review, the STents Versus AnGioplasty (STAG) trial.[3] Meta-analysis of both trials confirmed no improvement in technical success, patency, or clinical outcomes for primary stent placement over selective stenting. The authors concluded that the level of evidence was poor for recommendations, and they did not advocate primary stenting over selective stenting for symptomatic iliac disease.
- The UK National Institute for Health and Care Excellence (NICE) guidelines state, "Do not offer primary stent placement for treating people with intermittent claudication caused by aorto-iliac disease."[5]

Summary and Implications: This study suggests that patients undergoing iliac intervention (mostly CIA) for claudication should have a PTA with selective stenting approach. There is a high likelihood of technical success in the short term, with sustained patency into the medium and long term. It is important to counsel patients that around half will have persistent PAD symptoms in the long term, even with surgical intervention.

CLINICAL CASE: STENTING FOR ILIAC ARTERY DISEASE

Case History

A 54-year-old man comes to the vascular surgery outpatient clinic complaining of worsening pain in the right calf on walking. Over the last 6 months his pain-free walking distance has deteriorated from 500 yards to ~50 yards. He currently works as a postman but is increasingly struggling to complete his rounds. He is an ex-smoker but has no other comorbid illnesses. He sleeps at night with his legs in the bed and has never had any ulceration or gangrene in the foot. His general practitioner started him on clopidogrel and atorvastatin at the same time as referral, but despite starting these 8 weeks ago he hasn't noticed any symptomatic benefit. On examination he has a full complement of pulses in the left leg, but on the right he has a weak femoral pulse and nothing below. ABPI in the clinic is 0.7 on the right, which drops to 0.3 on exercise. Duplex ultrasonography in the clinic confirms a 3-cm-long >70% stenosis of the right CIA, with nonstenotic disease of the external iliac artery and patent arterial tree below. You order a computed tomographic (CT) angiogram to further characterize the iliac lesion. What is your next step?

Suggested Answer

For patients with intermittent claudication, the first steps should be to optimize medical therapy (e.g., stop smoking; start antiplatelet and high-dose statin therapy) as well as enroll them in a supervised exercise program. Here the patient has already stopped smoking and the general practitioner has initiated medical treatment with no symptomatic relief. It could be argued that the patient should now undergo supervised exercise therapy for 3 months prior to intervention. In this patient, however, this is unlikely to be successful: As a postman he walks a considerable distance every day as part of his rounds and will continue to do so in the near future. It would therefore be justified to offer intervention on the grounds that his symptoms are significantly impacting his quality of life and ability to work. According to the Dutch Iliac Stent Trial he should be offered primary PTA with the option of stenting if the stenosis is refractory to PTA. It is important to explain to the patient that he has a 50% chance of having PAD symptoms in the long term.

References

1. Klein QM, Van der Graaf Y, Seegers J, et al. Dutch Iliac Stent Trial: Long-term results in patients randomized for primary or selective stent placement. *Vasc Interv Radiol.* 2006;238(2):734–744.
2. Jongsma H, Bekken J, Ayez N, et al. Angioplasty versus stenting for iliac artery lesions. *Cochrane Database Syst Rev.* 2020;(12):CD007561.
3. Goode SD, Cleveland TJ, Gaines PA, STAG Trial Collaborators. Randomized clinical trial of stents versus angioplasty for the treatment of iliac artery occlusions (STAG trial). *Br J Surg.* 2013;100(9):1148–1153. DOI:10.1002/bjs.9197
4. Hajibandeh S, Hajibanndeh S, Antoniou SA, et al. Covered vs. uncovered stents for aortoiliac and femoropopliteal arterial disease: A systematic review and meta-analysis. *J Endovasc Ther.* 2016;23(3):442–452. DOI:10.1177/1526602816643834
5. National Institute of Health and Care Excellence Clinical Guideline 147. Peripheral arterial disease. https://www.nice.org.uk/Guidance/CG147

37

Risk of Death Following Application of Paclitaxel-Coated Balloons and Stents in the Femoropopliteal Artery of the Leg

A Systematic Review and Meta-analysis of Randomized Controlled Trials

> The potential causes of this alarming late increased incidence of death remain unknown.
>
> KATSANOS ET AL.

Research Question: Is there any increased risk of mortality with the use of paclitaxel-coated balloons and stents in the femoropopliteal artery?[1]

Funding: None

Year Range for Searches: 1964–2018

Year Study Published: 2018

Patients: 4,663

Which Studies Were Included: Randomized controlled study design investigating the use of a paclitaxel-coated/paclitaxel-eluting stent or balloon in the femoropopliteal artery for peripheral arterial disease (PAD) with an available follow-up of ≥1 year.

Which Studies Were Excluded: Case reports and observational or retrospective studies were excluded, as well as conference abstracts, editorials, and commentaries. Randomized controlled trials (RCTs) published with <1 year of follow-up were also excluded. Studies investigating paclitaxel treatment of below-the-knee arteries.

Study Overview: This was a meta-analysis to investigate the risk of death following the use of paclitaxel-coated balloons or stents in the femoropopliteal artery.

Study Intervention: A comprehensive search strategy was used to include terms for femoral artery, popliteal artery, femoropopliteal artery, balloon angioplasty, paclitaxel-eluting balloons, paclitaxel-coated balloons, paclitaxel-eluting stents, paclitaxel-coated stents, paclitaxel-eluting stents, drug-coated balloons, and drug-eluting stents.

Follow-up: Median RCT follow-up period was 2 years (range, 1–5 years).

Endpoints: Data extracted from each RCT included demographics, procedural variables, follow-up time period, prescribed antiplatelet therapy, and outcome data on patient mortality during different time periods. The main outcome measure was all-cause mortality.

RESULTS

- 28 RCTs were included involving a total of 4,663 patients. In four studies the intervention was drug-eluting stents and 24 studies used drug-coated balloons. Bias assessment (Cochrane Collaboration Tool) revealed overall low risk.
- The majority of included patients had intermittent claudication (89%), and two thirds of the participants were men. High rates of hypertension, diabetes mellitus, smoking, and hyperlipidemia were reported, with some heterogeneity within and between trials.
- There was no increased risk of all-cause death at 1 year for those patients receiving paclitaxel-impregnated device interventions compared to plain devices (risk ratio [RR] 1.08, 95% confidence interval [CI] 0.72–1.61) (all 28 studies included) (Table 37.1).
- 2-year data were available for 12 studies (2,316 patients). In these studies, patients undergoing treatment with paclitaxel devices had a significantly increased risk of all-cause mortality (RR 1.68, 95% CI 1.15–2.47); the

absolute death rate was 7.2% versus 3.8%, translating to a number needed to harm of 29 patients.
- At 5 years three studies were suitable for analysis (863 patients), and the increased mortality risk with the use of paclitaxel devices persisted (RR 1.93, 95% CI 1.27–2.93). In total 14.7% versus 8.1% of patients had died at 5 years in the paclitaxel group versus the control group, respectively.
- Excess risk of death per paclitaxel milligram year was calculated as 0.4 ± 0.1% (p = 0.001).

Table 37.1 SENSITIVITY AND SUBGROUP ANALYSES OF ALL-CAUSE DEATH

	RR (95% CI)
All-cause death at 2 years	1.68 (1.15–2.47)
All-cause death at 4-5 years	1.93 (1.27–2.93)
Paclitaxel drug-eluting stent only	1.87 (1.11–3.15)
Paclitaxel drug-coated balloon only	1.44 (1.04–2.00)
3.5 µg/mm² paclitaxel balloon	2.31 (1.15–4.63)
3.0 µg/mm² paclitaxel stent	2.10 (1.15–3.83)
3.0 µg/mm² paclitaxel balloon	1.65 (0.95–2.87)
2.0 µg/mm² paclitaxel balloon	1.27 (0.70–2.32)

Criticisms and Limitations: The studies included in this meta-analysis were not designed to investigate clinical outcomes (especially not mortality), making this a post-hoc analysis. In addition, causes of death were the crucial missing data in the studies that were analyzed; this information is necessary to determine whether there is causation or not.

Other Relevant Studies and Information

- When this analysis was published, three nationally funded PAD trials including drug-eluting (paclitaxel) devices (Swedish Drug-Elution Trials in Peripheral Arterial Disease [SWEDEPAD],[2] BAlloon Versus Stenting in Severe Ischemia of the Leg-3 [BASIL-3],[3] and Best Endovascular Versus Best Surgical Therapy for Patients with Critical Limb Ischemia [BEST-CLI][4]) paused recruitment while the UK Medicines and Healthcare Products Regulatory Agency (MHRA) and the US Food and Drug Administration (FDA) investigated the outcomes of the Katsanos et al. analysis. The MHRA removed the recommendation for use in patients with intermittent claudication but permitted use in selected patients with chronic limb-threatening ischemia and inside trials.[5] The FDA was more liberal, allowing their use when risks had been explained to patients and clinicians felt there were strong indications for their use.[6] Ultimately, all three of these trials resumed participant recruitment, and subsequent data on the risks of paclitaxel devices will be evaluated.

- Other meta-analyses assessing the safety of paclitaxel devices have had mixed results.[8,9]
- The Global Vascular Guideline has called for additional trials with long-term follow-up to further investigate the safety of paclitaxel devices.[10]

Summary and Implications: This meta-analysis of randomized trials involving the use of paclitaxel devices for the treatment of PAD in the femoropopliteal artery has raised concerns about excess mortality at 2 years and beyond. Further research into this concern is ongoing. In the meantime, paclitaxel devices for treating PAD should generally be avoided unless there is a compelling reason to use them.

CLINICAL CASE: ANGIOPLASTY OF THE SUPERFICIAL FEMORAL ARTERY

Case History

A 57-year-old man is in the clinic to discuss treatment of his intermittent claudication. You saw him 6 months previously and established best medical therapy (antiplatelet, atorvastatin, and smoking cessation) and enrolled him in your local supervised exercise program. He has valiantly controlled his comorbidities and for the most part attended his exercise program, but to no avail: He is still only able to walk 100 yards. He has a good femoral pulse but no pulses below; duplex ultrasonography reveals a 5-cm occlusion of the superficial femoral artery at the adductor hiatus. How should you proceed? What considerations are there, and how would you counsel the patient?

Suggested Answer

First, it is important to explain to the patient that currently his limb loss risk is very low. An option is to continue with conservative treatment and accept impaired walking as a lifestyle limitation. If the patient is not happy to pursue this strategy, he has the option of endovascular or surgical intervention. Most vascular surgeons would suggest an endovascular approach first in a Global Limb Anatomic Staging System (GLASS) stage 1 lesion of the femoropopliteal segment. Options here are plain balloon angioplasty with selective stenting, primary drug-coated balloons with selective stenting, primary drug-eluting stents, or primary covered stenting. Risks and benefits of each strategy should be discussed with the patient, including the large limitations regarding long-term outcome evidence with some of the devices. Excess mortality with drug-coated balloons/drug-eluting stents should also be relayed to the patient clearly. It would seem sensible not to use drug-coated balloons/drug-eluting stents primarily for a de novo chronic total occlusion, taking into account the results of this study.

References

1. Katsanos K, Spiliopoulos S, Kitrou P, et al. Risk of death following application of paclitaxel-coated balloons and stents in the femoropoliteal artery of the leg: A systematic review and meta-analysis of randomized controlled trials. *J Am Heart Assoc.* 2018;7(24):e011245. DOI:10.1161/JAHA.118.011245
2. Nordanstig J, Falkenberg M. The Swedish Drug-Elution Trials in Peripheral Arterial Disease (SWEDEPAD): An update halfway through the overall inclusion. *Eur J Vasc Endovasc Surg.* 2019;58(6):e367–e368.
3. Hunt BD, Popplewell MA, Davies H, et al. BAlloon versus Stenting in Severe Ischaemia of the Leg-3 (BASIL-3): Study protocol for a randomised controlled trial. *Trials.* 2017;18(1):224. doi:10.1186/s13063-017-1968-6
4. Menard MT, Farber A, Assmann SF, et al. Design and rationale of the Best Endovascular Versus Best Surgical Therapy for Patients with Critical Limb Ischemia (BEST-CLI) trial. *J Am Heart Assoc.* 2016;5(7):e003219. DOI:10.1161/JAHA.116.003219
5. UK Medicines and Healthcare Products Regulatory Agency. https://www.gov.uk/drug-device-alerts/paclitaxel-drug-coated-balloons-dcbs-or-drug-eluting-stents-dess-reconfirmed-position-on-use-in-patients-with-intermittent-claudication-and-critical-limb-ischaemia. Updated 2021.
6. US Food and Drug Administration. https://www.fda.gov/medical-devices/letters-health-care-providers/august-7-2019-update-treatment-peripheral-arterial-disease-paclitaxel-coated-balloons-and-paclitaxel. Updated 2021.
7. Nordanstig J, James S, Andersson M, et al. Mortality with paclitaxel-coated devices in peripheral artery disease. *N Engl J Med.* 2020;383:2438–2546. DOI:10.1056/NEJMoa2005206
8. Rocha-Singh KJ, Duval S, Jaff MR, et al. Mortality and paclitaxel-coated devices. *Circulation.* 2020;141(23):1859–1869.
9. Schneider PA, Laird JR, Doros G, et al. Mortality not correlated with paclitaxel exposure: An independent patient level meta-analysis of drug-coated balloon. *J Am Coll Cardiol.* 2019;72(20):2550–2563.
10. Conte MS, Bradbury AW, Kolh P, et al. Global vascular guidelines on the management of chronic limb-threatening ischemia. *J Vasc Surg.* 2019;69:3S–125S.

38

Meta-analysis of Open and Endovascular Repair of Popliteal Artery Aneurysms

> The overall literature is lacking in quality, and the need for well-controlled studies is critically important.
>
> LEAKE ET AL.

Research Question: What is the optimal treatment for the repair of popliteal artery aneurysms?[1]

Funding: None

Dates of Searches: 1994–2016

Year Study Published: 2017

Number of Studies Included in Systematic Review: 14 studies included in the meta-analysis

Which Studies Were Included: Included studies could be randomized controlled trials (RCTs) or cohort studies with a minimum of five patients in each group. The study needed to include both interventions, open (OPAR) and endovascular repair (EPAR).

Which Studies Were Excluded: Studies were excluded if they were editorials, opinion pieces, reports published as meeting abstracts only, and studies that did not contain data for the included outcomes. Interventions for non-aneurysmal indications (occlusive disease, trauma) were excluded.

Study Overview: This was a meta-analysis investigating the outcomes of open and endovascular repair of popliteal artery aneurysms. A comprehensive search strategy was used to include terms for popliteal, artery, and aneurysm.

Follow-up: Up to 3-year follow-up

Endpoints: *Primary outcome measures:* Primary and secondary patency rates at 1 year and 3 years. *Secondary outcome measures:* Complications, length of stay, reinterventions, amputations, and 30-day mortality.

RESULTS

- 14 studies were included for analysis (one RCT, two registries, and 11 retrospective case series). The Newcastle–Ottawa scale for quality indicated that 13 of the 14 studies were of low quality and one study (an RCT) was of medium quality.
- Patients in the OPAR group were significantly younger (73 vs. 75.7 years, p = 0.001). In terms of reported comorbidities there was no significant difference in rates of hyperlipidemia, hypertension, diabetes mellitus, chronic obstructive pulmonary disease, coronary artery disease, end-stage renal failure, or smoking status.
- Those undergoing OPAR were significantly more likely (p = 0.013) to have single-vessel runoff (37.1% vs. 22.8%). Patient undergoing OPAR were more likely to have a wound complication (odds ratio [OR] 5.1, p = 0.001) and a longer inpatient length of stay (OR 2.2, p = 0.001). They were, however, less likely to suffer thrombotic complications (OR 0.4, p = 0.019) or undergo re-intervention (OR 0.27, p = 0.001). There was no significant difference in limb salvage (OR 0.9, p = 0.791) (Table 38.1).

Table 38.1 PATENCY OF OPAR OUTPERFORMED EPAR AT 1 AND 3 YEARS

Patency	OPAR	EPAR	RR	p value
1-year primary patency	88.3%	81.2%	0.6	0.001
3-year primary patency	79.4%	68.2%	0.6	0.006
1-year secondary patency	92.3%	86.3%	0.8	0.57
3-year secondary patency	86.6%	80.0%	0.6	0.073

Criticisms and Limitations: There are no large RCTs trials on the topic, limiting the quality of studies included in this meta-analysis.

Other Relevant Studies and Information

- Current evidence (of low quality) supports that OPAR is a technically more robust solution for popliteal aneurysms reaching threshold for intervention. EPAR is more likely to occlude in the short and medium term, particularly when risk factors are present (e.g., acute ischemia, smaller-diameter stent-graft, longer stent-grafts, angulation of stent-graft, and poor outflow).[2,3]
- UK guidelines on EPAR indicate that it should only be performed after discussion with the multidisciplinary team and with special arrangements for clinical governance, consent, and audit in place[4] to carefully monitor short-term safety and long-term efficacy.
- The Society of Vascular Surgery guidelines for repair of popliteal aneurysms indicate that open repair is beneficial for patients with life expectancy of >5 years and a suitable venous conduit.[5]

Summary and Implications: This meta-analysis involving studies assessing the treatment of popliteal aneurysms with endovascular versus open approaches found that EPAR can be a safe and effective option in patients where OPAR is contraindicated. However, because there have not been any large RCTs comparing these treatment approaches, there is a need for ongoing research on this topic.

CLINICAL CASE: POPLITEAL ARTERY ANEURYSM

Case History

A 72-year-old man with popliteal artery aneurysm has been under surveillance since his abdominal aortic aneurysm was repaired 5 years ago. His most recent ultrasound scan has shown an increase in size to 2.8 cm, with thrombus lining the walls of the aneurysm. There is two-vessel runoff below the aneurysm and a healthy length of popliteal artery above and below the aneurysm. He currently has no compressive or occlusive symptoms and plays 18 holes of golf 2 days per week. What treatment if any would you recommend this patient have?

Suggested Answer

This patient's popliteal aneurysm has three indications for intervention: (1) >2 cm in diameter; (2) thrombus within the sac; and (3) loss of a tibial vessel below (may not be related). In terms of suitability for endovascular treatment, it is likely he is suitable as he has a length of popliteal artery above and below the aneurysm to land a stent (>15 mm is the recommendation). Given that the patient is still relatively active and survived an open abdominal aortic aneurysm repair 5 years prior, he is fit and would stand to lose quite a lot of function should his popliteal aneurysm occlude. Taking into account the results of this meta-analysis, the more durable option for this man would be OPAR; however, if it was his preference he could choose to undergo EPAR with the caveats mentioned above.

References

1. Leake AE, Segal MA, Chaer RA, et al. Meta-analysis of open endovascular repair of popliteal artery aneurysms. *J Vasc Surg.* 2017;65(1):246–256.
2. Crevin A, Acosta S, Hultgren R, et al. Results after open and endovascular repair of popliteal aneurysm: A matched comparison within a population-based cohort. *Eur J Vasc Endovasc Surg.* 2021;61(6):988–997. DOI:10.1016/j.ejves.2021.02.007
3. Zaghou MS, Andraska EA, Leake EA, et al. Poor runoff and distal coverage below the knee are associated with poor long-term outcomes following endovascular popliteal aneurysm repair. *J Vasc Surg.* 2021;74(1):153–160. DOI:10.1016/j.jvs.2020.12.062
4. National Institute for Health and Care Excellence. IPG 390: Endovascular stent-grafting of popliteal aneurysms. 2011. https://www.nice.org.uk/Guidance/IPG390
5. Faber A, Angle N, Avgerinos E, et al. The Society for Vascular Surgery clinical practice guidelines on popliteal artery aneurysms. *J Vasc Surg.* 2022;75(1):109–120.

39

A Prospective Study of Risk Factors for Diabetic Foot Ulcer

This study confirms important roles for neuropathy, Charcot deformity, skin oxygenation, larger vessel perfusion, body weight, past history of lower-limb complications, and poor vision in the etiology of diabetic foot ulcer.

BOYKO ET AL.

Research Question: What are the strongest risk factors for diabetic foot ulcers?[1]

Funding: None

Years Patients Were Treated: Not specified

Year Study Published: 1999

Study Location: Single clinical center from the United States.

Who Was Studied: All ambulatory patients with diabetes attending a general internal medicine clinic were eligible for enrollment.

Who Was Excluded: Exclusion criteria included current foot ulcer, bilateral foot amputations, wheelchair bound or unable to walk, too sick to participate, and psychiatric illness that prevented informed consent.

Patients: 749

Study Overview: This was a large prospective cohort study to assess the contributions of multiple factors to the risk of developing a diabetic foot ulcer.

Study Intervention: Patients were assessed for sensory and autonomic neuropathy as well as lower-limb transcutaneous oxygen tension $(TcPO_2)$, laser Doppler flowmetry, and ankle–brachial/toe pressure index (ABPI).

Follow-up: Mean follow-up of 3.7 years

Endpoints: The main outcome measure was the development of a foot ulcer, defined as a full-thickness skin defect that required >14 days to heal.

RESULTS

- This was a single-center study that recruited 749/900 consecutive patients (83.2%).
- The mean age of participants was 63.2 years. 98% were men (ex-army veterans). 93.6% had diabetes mellitus type 2; mean duration of diabetes was 11.4 years. 77% of patients completed follow-up, with a mean follow-up of 3.7 years.
- 162 ulcers developed in 5,442 person-years, giving an ulcer rate of 3.0/100 patient-years.
- Univariate Cox regression analysis indicated that 32 different factors contributed to the development of diabetic foot ulcer. When a multivariate analysis model was built to correct for traditional high-risk factors (sensory neuropathy, history of foot ulcer, history of amputation, insulin use, $TcPO_2$ dorsal foot, weight, Log ABPI, Charcot deformity, and vision <20/40), the only remaining risk factor to be significant was hammer/claw toes (Table 39.1).

Table 39.1 FACTORS SIGNIFICANTLY ASSOCIATED WITH FOOT ULCERATION
IN PATIENTS WITH DIABETES

	RR	95% CI	p value
Sensory neuropathy	2.17	1.52–3.08	<0.001
History of foot ulcer	1.63	1.17–2.26	0.004
History of amputation	2.81	1.84–4.29	<0.001
Insulin use	1.59	1.14–2.22	0.006
$TcPO_2$ dorsal foot	0.80	0.96–0.93	0.004
Weight	1.23	1.06–1.43	0.006
Log ABPI	0.83	0.73–0.96	0.011
Charcot deformity	3.49	1.22–9.92	0.019
Vision <20/40	1.93	1.42–2.63	<0.001
Hammer/claw toe	2.11	1.25–3.57	0.005

RR, Relative Risk; CI, confidence interval.

Criticisms and Limitations: Although this study identified risk factors correlated with the development of diabetic foot ulcers, as an observational analysis
it does not prove that any of these factors actually cause ulcers. Other factors be-
sides those assessed by the authors may have also been associated with diabetic
ulcer formation, such as prior receipt of surgical revascularization. The analysis also does not provide information on risk factors for ulcers requiring surgical intervention or amputation, nor on patient ambulation status throughout
the study.

Other Relevant Studies and Information: The myriad of associated factors for
the development of diabetic foot ulcer highlights the importance of multiple expertise in caring for these patients.[2,3] Clusters of triggers have been suggested to
start the process of diabetic foot ulcer, including (1) neuropathy, deformity, callus
formation, and elevated peak pressure; (2) peripheral vascular disease; (3) pene-
trating trauma; and (4) ill-fitting shoes. Tackling these clusters by ensuring the patient has good footwear, optimized circulation, appropriate eye care, and education
could help reduce the incidence of diabetic foot ulcer in 61% of patients.[4] Patient
education alone has not been found to have a significant impact in preventing diabetic foot ulcer in the long term.[5]

Summary and Implications: This study confirms many of the risk factors we
consider when assessing diabetic patients for the risks of developing foot ulceration. The most notable are sensory neuropathy, Charcot deformity, and history
of amputation. Unfortunately, many of the risk factors identified in this analysis
are difficult to modify.

CLINICAL CASE: DIABETIC FOOT ULCER

Case History
A 60-year-old diabetic woman presents to the multidisciplinary diabetic foot
clinic with a 3-week history of an ulcer at the proximal interphalangeal joint
(PIPJ) of the hallux on the left foot. She is known to have neuropathy with
clawing of the toes in both feet. She was moved on to insulin therapy 2 years ago
because of inadequate blood glucose control on oral treatment. Apart from the
ulcer she does describe some pain in the foot. On examination she has a very
good femoral pulse and high popliteal pulse but nothing below. She has audible,
incompressible monophasic Doppler signal at the dorsalis pedis. How do you
proceed?

Suggested Answer

It is likely this patient has a combination of neuropathic and ischemic ulceration. A full set of blood tests should be done to exclude systemic sepsis
from underlying osteomyelitis from the PIPJ of the hallux. She should undergo x-ray of the toes and the foot to look for more extensive osteomyelitis. The wound should be swabbed to target antimicrobial treatment. She
should be treated with empirical antibiotic treatment until the results from
the investigations are available. Her foot should be staged to define the underlying degree of limb threat (Wound, Ischemia and Foot Infection [WIfI]
score). In terms of the ischemic element, duplex ultrasonography and angiography should be performed with planned early revascularization as deemed appropriate (Global Limb Anatomic Staging System [GLASS] stage of anatomy
of disease). On admission the patient should be reviewed by a diabetologist
to ensure her treatment is optimized, and her vision should be tested to ex-
plore any potentially correctable visual impairment. It is likely this patient will
require minor amputation of the hallux to eradicate osteomyelitis. Once this
been performed, she should be assessed by the inpatient podiatric service for
adequate off-loading footwear in both feet. Patient education regarding foot
care should be an ongoing process during her admission and reinforced when
she is discharged and followed up closely in the outpatient diabetic foot clinic.

References

1. Boyko EJ, Ahroni JH, Stensel V, et al. A prospective study of risk factor for diabetic
   foot ulcer. *Diabetes Care.* 1999;22:1036–1042.
2. Buggy A, Moore Z. The impact of the multidisciplinary team in the management of individuals with diabetic foot ulcers: A systematic review. *J Wound Care.*
   2017;26(6):324–339.
3. Huizing E, Schreve MA, Kortmann W, et al. The effect of a multidisciplinary outpatient team approach on outcomes in diabetic foot care: A single-center study. *J
   Cardiovasc Surg.* 2019;60(6):662–671.
4. Lavery LA, Peters EJG, Armstrong DA. What are the most effective interventions in
   preventing diabetic foot ulcers? *Int Wound J.* 2008;5(3):425–433.
5. Dorresteijn JAN, Kriegsman DMW, Assendelft WJJ, Valk GD. Patient education for
   preventing diabetic foot ulceration. *Cochrane Database Syst Rev.* 2012;10:CD001488.

Venous Disease

JULIEN AL SHAKARCHI AND ISAAC NYAMEKYE

40

Long-Term Outcome After Additional Catheter-Directed Thrombolysis Versus Standard Treatment for Acute Iliofemoral Deep Vein Thrombosis (the CaVenT Study)

A Randomized Controlled Trial

Additional [catheter-directed thrombolysis] improved the clinically relevant long-term outcome after iliofemoral [deep venous thrombosis] by reducing [post-thrombotic syndrome].

THE CAVENT INVESTIGATORS[1]

Research Question: Does catheter-directed thrombolysis (CDT) for iliofemoral deep vein thrombosis (DVT) reduce the occurrence of post-thrombotic syndrome (PTS)?

Funding: South-Eastern Norway Regional Health Authority; Research Council of Norway; University of Oslo; Oslo University Hospital

Year Study Began: 2006

Year Study Published: 2012

Study Location: 20 clinical centers in Norway

Who Was Studied: Inclusion criteria were:
- Age 18–75 years
- Onset of symptoms within the past 21 days
- Objectively verified (by diagnostic imaging) DVT localized in the upper half of the thigh, the common iliac vein, or the combined iliofemoral segment
- Informed consent

Who Was Excluded: Patients were excluded if they had received anticoagulant treatment before trial entry for more than the past 7 days or any thrombolytic treatment within 7 days before trial inclusion, had a contraindication to thrombolytic treatment, had another indication for thrombolytic treatment, or had any severe condition such as anemia, renal failure, history of subarachnoid or intracerebral bleeding, or any condition with a life expectancy <24 months.

Patients: 209

Study Overview

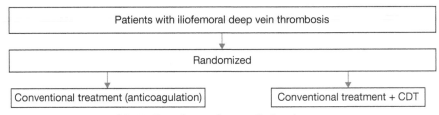

Figure 40.1 Design of CaVenT randomized controlled trial

Study Intervention: In this randomized controlled trial (RCT), patients were randomly assigned to conventional treatment with anticoagulation, or to CDT in addition to anticoagulation.

Follow-up: Duration of follow-up was 24 months.

Endpoints: *Primary outcome measures:* Iliofemoral patency after 6 months and frequency of PTS after 24 months. *Secondary outcome measures:* Frequency of clinically relevant bleeding related to CDT, recurrent venous thromboembolism (VTE) during follow-up, and PTS at 6 months.

RESULTS

- Mean age was 51.5 years (standard deviation [SD] 15.8) and 37% of participants were female. Mean duration of symptoms was 6.6 days (SD 4.6). For those receiving CDT, mean duration of treatment was 2.4 days (SD 1.1).
- At 24 months of follow-up, the proportion of patients still on oral anticoagulation with an International Normalized Ratio (INR) within the therapeutic range (2.0–3.0) was 65.4% (95% confidence interval [CI] 46.2–80.6) in the CDT group versus 50.0% (95% CI 32.1–67.9) of those in the control group. At 24 months of follow-up, 63.3% (95% CI 53.3–72.6) in the CDT group reported daily use of elastic compression stockings compared with 51.5% (95% CI 41.2–61.2) in the control group (Table 40.1).
- Iliofemoral patency after 6 months was significantly higher in the CDT group (65.9% [55.5–75.0]) compared with the control group (47.4% [37.6–57.3]) and the frequency of PTS after 24 months was significantly lower in the CDT group (41.1% [31.5–51.4]) compared with the control group (55.6% [45.7–65.0]).
- 20 bleeding complications related to CDT included three major and five clinically relevant bleeds. During follow-up, 28 patients had recurrent VTE and 11 were diagnosed with cancer; there was no significant difference between the groups.

Table 40.1 SHORT- AND LONG-TERM OUTCOMES

	CDT group	Medical group	p value
PTS at 24 months	37 (41.1%)	55 (55.6%)	0.047
Iliofemoral patency at 6 months	58 (65.9%)	45 (47.4%)	0.012
PTS at 6 months	27 (30.3%)	32 (32.2%)	0.77

Criticisms and Limitations

- Due to loss to follow-up, the final study population was closer to the critical limit for detection of a clinical effect and the effect estimate was imprecise according to the authors.

- Another limitation of the study included possible differences in the interventions carried out by the interventional centers. In addition, current advocates of deep venous interventions will argue that newer technology is now available that would further improve the results.

Other Relevant Studies and Information

- The UK National Institute for Health and Care Excellence (NICE) guideline states that for acute iliofemoral DVT, the evidence on efficacy for percutaneous mechanical thrombectomy is limited in quality and quantity; therefore, this procedure should only be used with special arrangements for clinical governance, consent, and audit or research.[2]
- The Society for Vascular Surgery suggests the use of early thrombus-removal strategies in ambulatory patients with good functional capacity and a first episode of iliofemoral DVT of <14 days in duration and strongly recommend their use in patients with limb-threatening ischemia due to iliofemoral venous outflow obstruction.[3]
- Following this landmark paper, two further RCTs have been published and will be discussed in Chapter 41: the Acute Venous Thrombosis: Thrombus Removal with Adjunctive Catheter-Directed Thrombolysis (ATTRACT)[4] trial and the Ultrasound-Accelerated Catheter-Directed Thrombolysis on Preventing Post-Thrombotic Syndrome (CAVA)[5] trial.

Summary and Implications: For patients with iliofemoral DVT, CDT improved PTS compared with conventional treatment with anticoagulation and elastic compression stockings alone. This improvement was at a cost of a small additional risk of bleeding. Major guidelines currently recommend consideration of CDT in carefully selected patients with iliofemoral DVT at high risk for PTS and low risk for procedure-related complications. Further studies of CDT in the treatment of DVT are ongoing.

CLINICAL CASE: EXTENSIVE ILIOFEMORAL DVT

Case History

A 25-year-old woman presents to the emergency department with acute-onset pain and swelling in her right leg. She has recently come back from China on a long-haul flight. She is otherwise fit and well. A duplex ultrasound confirms an extensive iliofemoral DVT. After 48 hours of leg elevation and anticoagulation, her leg is still very swollen and she is only able to mobilize for a few steps. How would you manage this patient?

Suggested Answer

This patient has an extensive symptomatic iliofemoral DVT that has not responded to medical management. Following a multidisciplinary team discussion and a comprehensive consent process, she undergoes successful CDT. This improves her symptoms and she is discharged fully mobile within a few days of the procedure.

References

1. Enden T, Haig Y, Kløw NE, et al. Long-term outcome after additional catheter-directed thrombolysis versus standard treatment for acute iliofemoral deep vein thrombosis (the CaVenT study): A randomised controlled trial. *Lancet.* 2012;379(9810):31–38.
2. National Institute for Health and Care Excellence (NICE). Percutaneous mechanical thrombectomy for acute deep vein thrombosis of the leg. 2019. https://www.nice.org.uk/guidance/IPG651
3. Meissner MH, Gloviczki P, Comerota AJ, et al. Early thrombus removal strategies for acute deep venous thrombosis: Clinical practice guidelines of the Society for Vascular Surgery and the American Venous Forum. *J Vasc Surg.* 2012;55(5):1449–1462.
4. Vedantham S, Goldhaber SZ, Julian JA, et al. Pharmacomechanical catheter-directed thrombolysis for deep-vein thrombosis. *N Engl J Med.* 2017;377(23):2240–2252.
5. Notten P, de Smet AAEA, Tick LW, et al. CAVA (Ultrasound-Accelerated Catheter-Directed Thrombolysis on Preventing Post-Thrombotic Syndrome) trial: Long-term follow-up results. *J Am Heart Assoc.* 2021;10(11):e018973.

41

Pharmacomechanical Catheter-Directed Thrombolysis for Deep Vein Thrombosis

The Acute Venous Thrombosis: Thrombus Removal with Adjunctive Catheter-Directed Thrombolysis (ATTRACT) Trial

In this trial, pharmacomechanical thrombolysis did not prevent the post-thrombotic syndrome in patients with acute proximal deep vein thrombosis.

THE ATTRACT INVESTIGATORS

Research Question: Does pharmacomechanical thrombolysis for deep vein thrombosis (DVT) reduce the risk of post-thrombotic syndrome (PTS)?[1]

Funding: National Heart, Lung, and Blood Institute of the National Institutes of Health, Boston Scientific, Covidien (now Medtronic), Genentech and BSN Medical

Year Study Began: 2009

Year Study Published: 2017

Study Location: 56 clinical centers in the US

Who Was Studied: Inclusion criteria were:
- Symptomatic proximal DVT involving the femoral, common femoral, or iliac vein (with or without other involved ipsilateral veins)
- Onset of symptoms within 14 days

Who Was Excluded:
Exclusion criteria were:

- <16 or >75 years of age
- Pregnant
- At high bleeding risk
- Active cancer
- Established PTS
- Ipsilateral DVT in the previous 2 years

Patients: 692

Study Overview

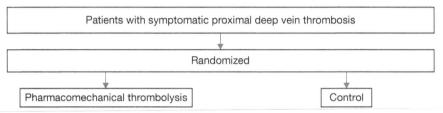

Figure 41.1 Design of ATTRACT randomized controlled trial

Study Intervention: In this randomized controlled trial (RCT), patients were randomly assigned to the pharmacomechanical-thrombolysis group or the control group (no procedural intervention).

Follow-up: Follow-up period of 24 months

Endpoints: *Primary outcome measures:* Development of PTS between the 6-month follow-up visit and the 24-month visit. *Secondary outcome measures:* The occurrence of PTS at 6, 12, 18, and 24 months, moderate to severe PTS, major bleeding, and recurrent venous thromboembolism (VTE).

RESULTS

- Within 7 days after randomization, five patients who had been assigned to the control group underwent pharmacomechanical thrombolysis and 11 patients who had been assigned to the pharmacomechanical-thrombolysis group did not undergo the procedure. These patients were excluded from the per-protocol analysis.

- Between 6 and 24 months, there was no significant between-group difference in the percentage of patients with PTS (47% in the pharmacomechanical-thrombolysis group and 48% in the control group; risk ratio [RR], 0.96; 95% confidence interval [CI], 0.82–1.11; p = 0.56) (Table 41.1).
- Moderate to severe PTS occurred in 18% of patients in the pharmacomechanical-thrombolysis group versus 24% of those in the control group (RR, 0.73; 95% CI, 0.54–0.98; p = 0.04).
- Pharmacomechanical thrombolysis led to more major bleeding events within 10 days (1.7% vs. 0.3% of patients, p = 0.049), but no significant difference in recurrent VTE was seen over the 24-month follow-up period (12% in the pharmacomechanical-thrombolysis group and 8% in the control group, p = 0.09).

Table 41.1 Trial outcomes

Outcome	Pharmacomechanical-thrombolysis group (n = 336)	Control group (n = 355)	p value
PTS	157 (47%)	171 (48%)	0.56
Moderate to severe PTS	60 (18%)	84 (24%)	0.04
Major bleeding, first 10 days	6 (1.7%)	1 (0.3%)	0.049
Recurrent VTE over 24 months	42 (12%)	30 (8%)	0.09

Criticisms and Limitations

- The main criticism of the study was the inclusion of femoral DVT in the study. Generally these patients have always been treated with medical management and their inclusion was controversial.
- Another criticism of the study was that there was a substantial number of missing assessments of PTS. In addition, a large number of patients had to be screened in order to enroll the target sample, and this therefore might reduce the generalizability of the trial.
- There was also variation in how the pharmacomechanical-thrombolysis procedure was performed, in order to accommodate patient-specific differences and physician preferences.
- Most patients received warfarin; although direct oral anticoagulants are now frequently used, the effect of this on PTS rates is unknown.

Other Relevant Studies and Information

- The Ultrasound-Accelerated Catheter-Directed Thrombolysis on Preventing Post-Thrombotic Syndrome (CAVA) trial was a multicenter RCT conducted in 15 hospitals in the Netherlands assessing ultrasound-accelerated catheter-directed thrombolysis versus medical treatment for acute iliofemoral DVT. In this study, the impact of additional ultrasound-accelerated catheter-directed thrombolysis on the prevention of PTS was found to increase with time.[2]
- The UK National Institute for Health and Care Excellence (NICE) guideline states that for acute iliofemoral DVT, the evidence on efficacy for percutaneous-mechanical thrombectomy is limited in quality and quantity; therefore, this procedure should only be used with special arrangements for clinical governance, consent, and audit or research.[3]
- The European Society for Vascular Surgery guidelines recommend that early thrombus-removal strategies should be considered in selected patients with symptomatic iliofemoral DVT.[4]

Summary and Implications: Among patients with acute proximal DVT, the addition of pharmacomechanical catheter-directed thrombolysis to anticoagulation did not result in a lower risk of PTS but did result in a higher risk of major bleeding.

CLINICAL CASE: ILIOFEMORAL DVT

Case History
A 60-year-old man presents to the emergency department with acute-onset pain and swelling in his left leg. He has recently had a knee replacement on the contralateral side. He is otherwise medically well apart from suffering from hypertension. A duplex ultrasound confirms an iliofemoral DVT. How would you manage this patient?

Suggested Answer
This patient has a symptomatic iliofemoral DVT and needs to be started on anticoagulation. After 72 hours of leg elevation and anticoagulation, his leg is less swollen and he is able to mobilize. In view of the improvement in his symptoms, he does not require any invasive intervention.

References

1. Vedantham S, Goldhaber SZ, Julian JA, et al. Pharmacomechanical catheter-directed thrombolysis for deep-vein thrombosis. *N Engl J Med.* 2017;377(23):2240–2252.
2. Notten P, de Smet AAEA, Tick LW, et al. CAVA (Ultrasound-Accelerated Catheter-Directed Thrombolysis on Preventing Post-Thrombotic Syndrome) trial: Long-term follow-up results. *J Am Heart Assoc.* 2021;10(11):e018973.
3. National Institute for Health and Care Excellence (NICE). Percutaneous mechanical thrombectomy for acute deep vein thrombosis of the leg. 2019. https://www.nice.org.uk/guidance/IPG651
4. Kakkos SK, Gohel M, Baekgaard N, et al. European Society for Vascular Surgery (ESVS) 2021 clinical practice guidelines on the management of venous thrombosis. *Eur J Vasc Endovasc Surg.* 2021;61(1):9–82.

42

Long-Term Results of Compression Therapy Alone Versus Compression Plus Surgery in Chronic Venous Ulceration

The Effect of Surgery and Compression on Healing and Recurrence (ESCHAR) Study, a Randomized Controlled Trial

> Surgical correction can . . . reduce the chance of recurrent ulceration and increase ulcer-free time.
>
> THE ESCHAR INVESTIGATORS

Research Question: Can recurrence of leg ulcers be prevented by surgical correction of superficial venous reflux in addition to compression?[1]

Funding: NHS Executive South and West Research and Development Directorate, Southmead Hospital Research Foundation, and Medical Research Council

Year Study Began: 1999

Year Study Published: 2007

Study Location: Three clinical centers in the UK

Who Was Studied: Inclusion criteria were:

- Open or recently healed leg ulceration (within 6 months) between knee and malleoli of >4 weeks' duration
- Ankle–brachial pressure index (ABPI) of ≥0.85
- Superficial or deep venous reflux on duplex scanning

Who Was Excluded: Exclusion criteria were:
- Duplex scanning not possible
- Multilayer compression therapy not practical
- Unable or unwilling to give informed consent
- Deep venous occlusion
- Unfit for surgery (even under local anesthetic)
- Malignant ulceration

Patients: 500

Study Overview

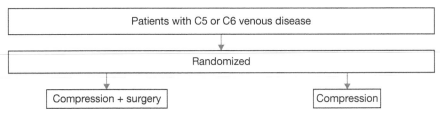

Figure 42.1 Design of ESCHAR randomized controlled trial

Study Intervention: In this randomized controlled trial, patients were randomly assigned to treatment with multilayer compression therapy alone or compression plus superficial open venous surgery.

Follow-up: 3 years of follow-up

Endpoints: *Primary outcome measures:* Ulcer healing (defined as complete re-epithelialization) and ulcer recurrence. *Secondary outcome measure:* Ulcer-free time (defined as the total time with a healed leg)

RESULTS

- Of 242 patients randomized to compression + surgery, 195 (81%) underwent the operation; surgery was carried out to the great saphenous vein in 141 (72%), the short saphenous vein in 27 (14%), and both the great and the small saphenous veins in 21 (11%).

- Ulcer healing rates at 3 years were 89% for the compression group and 93% for the compression + surgery group (p = 0.73, log rank test). Rates of ulcer recurrence at 4 years were 56% for the compression group and 31% for the compression + surgery group (p < 0.01).
- Recurrence rates were found to be significantly lower in the surgical group for patients with isolated superficial reflux only and isolated superficial reflux with segmental deep reflux.
- Patients in the compression + surgery group experienced a greater proportion of ulcer-free time after 3 years compared with patients in the compression group (78% vs. 71%; p = 0.007, Mann-Whitney U test).

Criticisms and Limitations

- The biggest limitation of the ESCHAR study is that it was not designed to assess healing; about one third of recruits had recently healed ulcers, and therefore the study was underpowered to assess ulcer healing.
- 24% of patients randomized to surgery did not undergo their operation despite extensive counseling before recruitment.
- Patients waited a median of 7 weeks for their operation and therefore may not have received an immediate benefit.
- For frailty reasons, many older patients had junctional ligation under local anesthesia rather an attempt to ablate all sources of incompetence.
- Class 2 stockings have been shown to reduce ulcer recurrence, but the study did not include a formal assessment of compliance with stocking use.

Other Relevant Studies and Information

- The 2015 European Society for Vascular Surgery guidelines on management of chronic venous disease recommend that compression should be used as the initial treatment modality for venous leg ulcers and active venous intervention should be explored and offered to maintain healing.[2]
- The 2014 Society for Vascular Surgery and American Venous Forum guidelines suggest ablation of the incompetent veins in addition to standard compressive therapy to improve ulcer healing and prevent recurrence.[3]
- Following this landmark paper, a further randomized controlled trial (the Early Venous Reflux Ablation [EVRA] trial)[4] has now been published and will be discussed in Chapter 43.

Summary and Implications: Among patients with chronic venous leg ulcerations and venous reflux on duplex scanning, the ESCHAR study found that superficial venous surgery in addition to compression reduced the risk of recurrence and increased ulcer-free time. The study did not show a significant improvement in wound healing rates. These results provide support for the provision of duplex scanning and superficial venous surgery for patients with chronic venous leg ulcers.

CLINICAL CASE: HEALED VENOUS ULCERATION

Case History
A 76-year-old woman attends your clinic with a recent history of an ulcer on her right lower leg. She recalls having a similar ulcer a few years ago, which healed with regular district nurse dressings. This time, she was again managed in the community with compression, and after 6 weeks the ulcer has now healed. The ultrasound duplex examination confirms an incompetent great saphenous vein with a patent and competent deep system. How would you manage this patient?

Suggested Answer
This patient has significant venous disease (C5), which led to the ulcer. Even though it has now healed, she should be considered for long-term management to avoid recurrence. As per the ESCHAR trial, she should be offered surgical intervention in addition to compression to decrease her risk of ulcer recurrence.

References

1. Gohel MS, Barwell JR, Taylor M, et al. Long-term results of compression therapy alone versus compression plus surgery in chronic venous ulceration (ESCHAR): Randomised controlled trial. *BMJ*. 2007;335(7610):83.
2. Wittens C, Davies AH, Bækgaard N, et al. Management of chronic venous disease: Clinical practice guidelines of the European Society for Vascular Surgery. *Eur J Vasc Endovasc Surg*. 2015;49(6):678–737.
3. O'Donnell TF Jr, Passman MA, Marston WA, et al. Management of venous leg ulcers: Clinical practice guidelines of the Society for Vascular Surgery and the American Venous Forum. *J Vasc Surg*. 2014;60(2 Suppl):3S–59S.
4. Gohel MS, Heatley F, Liu X, et al. A randomized trial of early endovenous ablation in venous ulceration. *N Engl J Med*. 2018;378(22):2105–2114.

43

A Randomized Trial of Early Endovenous Ablation in Venous Ulceration

The Early Venous Reflux Ablation (EVRA) Trial

We found that faster ulcer healing can be attained if an endovenous intervention is performed promptly.

THE EVRA INVESTIGATORS

Research Question: Can recurrence of leg ulcers be prevented by surgical correction of superficial venous reflux in addition to compression?[1]

Funding: National Institute for Health Research Health Technology Assessment Programme

Year Study Began: 2013

Year Study Published: 2018

Study Location: 20 clinical centers in the UK

Who Was Studied: Inclusion criteria were:
- Age >18 years
- Open venous leg ulcer that had been present for 6 weeks to 6 months
- Ankle–brachial pressure index (ABPI) of ≥0.8
- Primary or recurrent superficial venous reflux

Who Was Excluded: Exclusion criteria were:
- Pregnant
- Unable to adhere to compression therapy
- Deep venous occlusive disease or any other condition precluding superficial venous ablation
- Leg ulcers for which the cause was deemed to be non-venous or were thought to require skin grafting[1]

Patients: 450

Study Overview

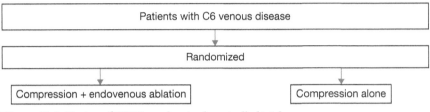

Figure 43.1 Design of EVRA randomized controlled trial

Study Intervention: In this randomized controlled trial, patients were randomly assigned to treatment with multilayer compression therapy alone or compression plus superficial endovenous ablation.

Follow-up: 3 years of follow-up

Endpoints: *Primary outcome measures:* Time to ulcer healing from the date of randomization through 12 months. *Secondary outcome measures:* Rate of ulcer healing at 24 weeks, rate of ulcer recurrence, length of time free from ulcers (ulcer-free time) during the first year after randomization, and patient-reported health-related quality of life.

RESULTS

- Patient and clinical characteristics at baseline were similar in the two treatment groups.
- The time to ulcer healing was shorter in the early-intervention group than in the deferred-intervention group; more patients had healed ulcers with early intervention (hazard ratio for ulcer healing, 1.38; 95% confidence interval [CI], 1.13–1.68; p = 0.001).

- The median time to ulcer healing was 56 days (95% CI, 49–66) in the early-intervention group and 82 days (95% CI, 69–92) in the deferred-intervention group.
- The rate of ulcer healing at 24 weeks was 85.6% in the early-intervention group and 76.3% in the deferred-intervention group.
- The median ulcer-free time during the first year after trial enrollment was 306 days (interquartile range, 240–328) in the early-intervention group and 278 days (interquartile range, 175–324) in the deferred-intervention group (p = 0.002).
- The most common procedural complications of endovenous ablation were pain and deep vein thrombosis.

Criticisms and Limitations

- All the recruitment centers had an established pathway of care for leg ulcers, and considerable variation existed among them. The centers used different surgical treatment protocols and methods of endovenous therapy, limiting insight on optimal treatment.
- >6,500 patients were screened to reach the target sample size of 450. Patients were often not eligible for inclusion in the trial because the ulcer had been present for >6 months or had already healed by the time of randomization. This may limit the generalizability of the EVRA findings in real-world practice.
- Variations were noted in the superficial veins that were refluxing and the presence and extent of deep venous reflux. However, findings from the current trial support other data showing that the clinical benefits of treating superficial venous reflux can be attained even in the presence of concomitant deep venous reflux.

Other Relevant Studies and Information

- The European Society for Vascular Surgery guidelines recommend that compression should be used as the initial treatment modality for venous leg ulcers and active venous intervention should be explored and offered to maintain healing.[2]
- The Society for Vascular Surgery and American Venous Forum guidelines suggest ablation of the incompetent veins in addition to standard compressive therapy to improve ulcer healing and prevent recurrence.[3]

Summary and Implications: Early endovenous ablation of superficial venous reflux resulted in faster healing of venous leg ulcers and more time free from ulcers than deferred endovenous ablation. This was found to be significant even though the rate of healing from the control group (compression) was outstanding and the best reported in the literature.

CLINICAL CASE: ACTIVE NEW-ONSET VENOUS ULCERATION

Case History

An 81-year-old retired butcher attends your clinic with a history of a ulcer on his left lower leg that started 3 weeks ago. He has been managed in the community, where personnel have confirmed palpable pulses and a reasonable ABPI (0.9) with regular dressings. The ultrasound duplex examination confirms an incompetent long saphenous vein and all other veins are patent and competent. How would you manage this patient?

Suggested Answer

This patient has an incompetent long saphenous vein and a venous ulcer. His ABPI is 0.95, and compression is started for him from clinic. As per the EVRA trial, he is offered endovenous ablation as soon as possible to promote ulcer healing and decrease his risk of ulcer recurrence.

References

1. Gohel MS, Heatley F, Liu X, et al. A randomized trial of early endovenous ablation in venous ulceration. *N Engl J Med.* 2018;378(22):2105–2114.
2. Wittens C, Davies AH, Bækgaard N, et al. Management of chronic venous disease: Clinical practice guidelines of the European Society for Vascular Surgery. *Eur J Vasc Endovasc Surg.* 2015;49(6):678–737.
3. O'Donnell TF Jr, Passman MA, Marston WA, et al. Management of venous leg ulcers: Clinical practice guidelines of the Society for Vascular Surgery and the American Venous Forum. *J Vasc Surg.* 2014;60(2 Suppl):3S–59S.

44

5-Year Outcomes of a Randomized Trial of Treatments for Varicose Veins

The Comparison of Laser, Surgery, and Foam Sclerotherapy (CLASS) Trial

[Aberdeen Varicose Vein Questionnaire] scores were better among participants treated with laser ablation or surgery than among those treated with foam sclerotherapy.

THE CLASS INVESTIGATORS

Research Question: Which treatment modality for varicose veins offers the best improvement in quality of life (QoL) and is the most cost-effective?[1]

Funding: National Institute for Health Research

Year Study Began: 2008

Year Study Published: 2019

Study Location: 11 clinical centers in the UK

Who Was Studied: Inclusion criteria were (1) age ≥18 years and (2) presence of primary symptomatic varicose veins (>3 mm in diameter) in one or both legs (more severely affected leg was designated as the study leg), and reflux of the great saphenous or small saphenous veins of >1 second as measured by duplex ultrasonography.

Who Was Excluded: Exclusion criteria were:
- Active deep vein thrombosis
- Acute superficial vein thrombosis
- Diameter of the main truncal saphenous vein of <3 mm or >15 mm
- Tortuous veins considered to be unsuitable for laser treatment
- Contraindications to the use of foam or to general or regional anesthesia

Patients: 798

Study Overview

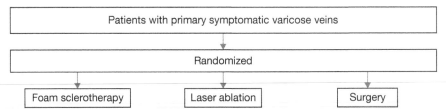

Figure 44.1 Design of CLASS randomized controlled trial

Study Intervention: In this randomized controlled trial, patients were randomly assigned to foam sclerotherapy, laser ablation (with subsequent foam sclerotherapy for residual varicosities, if necessary), or surgery.

Follow-up: 5-year analysis

Endpoints: *Primary outcome measures:* Participant-reported disease-specific QoL measured with the Aberdeen Varicose Vein Questionnaire (AVVQ), participant-reported generic QoL, and 5-year cost-effectiveness calculated as cost per quality-adjusted life-year (QALY) gained. *Secondary outcome measures:* QoL measured with the EQ-5D visual analog scale, clinical success as measured by the presence of varicose veins assessed by the participant and nurse using a visual analog scale and the Venous Clinical Severity Score, additional procedures for treatment of varicose veins, participant satisfaction and willingness to repeat and recommend the treatment.

RESULTS

- QoL questionnaires were completed by 595 (75%) of the 798 trial participants.
- After adjustment for baseline scores and other covariates, AVVQ scores (possible scores range from 0 to 100, with lower scores indicating a better QoL) were significantly lower among patients who underwent laser ablation (17.7 at baseline to 8.6 at 5 years) or surgery (18.3 at baseline to 8.7 at 5 years) than among those who underwent foam sclerotherapy (17.3 at baseline to 11 at 5 years).
- Generic QoL measures and EQ-5D visual analog scale scores did not differ among treatment groups.
- At a threshold willingness-to-pay ratio of £20,000 ($28,433 in US dollars) per QALY, 77.2% of the cost-effectiveness model iterations favored laser ablation. In a two-way comparison between foam sclerotherapy and surgery, 54.5% of the model iterations favored surgery.
- With regard to patient satisfaction, the majority of participants were willing to repeat the same treatment and to recommend the treatment they had received to a friend.
- The rates of complete truncal vein ablation at 5 years were 64.0% with laser ablation, 33.3% with foam sclerotherapy, and 75.9% with surgery.

Criticisms and Limitations

- Limitations of the study include the lack of a sham procedure and the lack of blinding as both patients and assessors were aware of the treatments.
- There was a substantial amount of missing data at 5 years, although the response rate with respect to participant-reported outcomes was high.
- The CLASS trial did not include a radiofrequency ablation arm, which has been shown to have slightly improved outcomes in other studies, and did not study more novel methods such as mechanochemical endovenous ablation.
- Another limitation of the trial is that patients with tortuous truncal veins or recurrent veins were excluded, and foam sclerotherapy may have had advantages for these patients. Also, the methodology of foam sclerotherapy used has been criticized by expert phlebologists as the technique and dosages were not optimal in a trial performed by UK vascular surgeons.

Other Relevant Studies and Information

- The UK National Institute for Health and Care Excellence (NICE) guidelines recommend first offering endothermal ablation treatment of the long saphenous vein, followed by ultrasound-guided foam sclerotherapy and finally open surgery.[2]
- The European Society for Vascular Surgery recommends the use of endovenous thermal ablation techniques over foam sclerotherapy and open surgery.[3]
- The Society for Vascular Surgery states that endovenous thermal ablations (laser and radiofrequency ablations) are safe and effective, and recommends their use for treatment of saphenous incompetence. They recommend endovenous thermal ablation of the incompetent saphenous vein over open surgery due to reduced convalescence and less pain and morbidity.[4]

Summary and Implications: In a randomized trial of three different treatments for symptomatic primary truncal saphenous varicose veins, disease-specific QoL 5 years after treatment was better after laser ablation or surgery than after foam sclerotherapy. The cost-effectiveness models showed laser ablation to be the most cost-effective at a willingness-to-pay ratio of £20,000 ($28,433) per QALY.

CLINICAL CASE: MANAGEMENT OF PRIMARY SMALL SAPHENOUS VEIN INCOMPETENCE

Case History

A 55-year-old male shop assistant is referred to your clinic with symptomatic primary varicose veins. He complains of generalized leg discomfort and mild ankle swelling, especially at the end of a long day at work. On examination, he has varicosities in the small saphenous vein distribution and the duplex ultrasound examination confirms an incompetence of the saphenopopliteal junction and the proximal 25 cm of the small saphenous vein (SSV). The incompetent SSV is straight and subfascial and suitable for open or endovenous therapy. How would this study help you in managing this patient?

Suggested Answer

The CLASS trial showed that there was no significant difference in ablation rates between open surgery and endovenous laser technique. However, there was a lower ablation rate with foam sclerotherapy. QoL scores also showed an advantage with both laser ablation and open surgery over foam sclerotherapy. The cost analysis within a UK National Health Service model suggested laser ablation to be the most cost-effective, and this should be offered to this patient. However, foam sclerotherapy in most settings is inexpensive, and even after several retreatments over time, might still be the least expensive option.

References

1. Brittenden J, Cooper D, Dimitrova M, et al. Five-year outcomes of a randomized trial of treatments for varicose veins. *N Engl J Med.* 2019;381(23):2275–2276.
2. National Institute for Health and Care Excellence (NICE). Varicose veins: Diagnosis and management. 2013. https://www.nice.org.uk/Guidance/CG168
3. Wittens C, Davies AH, Bækgaard N, et al. Management of chronic venous disease: Clinical practice guidelines of the European Society for Vascular Surgery. *Eur J Vasc Endovasc Surg.* 2015;49(6):678–737.
4. Gloviczki P, Comerota AJ, Dalsing MC, et al. The care of patients with varicose veins and associated chronic venous diseases: Clinical practice guidelines of the Society for Vascular Surgery and the American Venous Forum. *Vasc Surg.* 2011;53(5 Suppl):2S–48S.

45

Comparison of Endovenous Ablation Techniques, Foam Sclerotherapy, and Surgical Stripping for Great Saphenous Varicose Veins

Extended 5-Year Follow-up of a Randomized Controlled Trial

> Significantly more patients in the [ultrasound-guided foam sclero-therapy] group developed recanalization in the [great saphenous vein], compared with the other groups.
>
> LAWAETZ ET AL.

Research Question: Which treatment modality for varicose veins offers the best long-term clinical outcome?[1]

Funding: Public Health Insurance Research Foundation of Denmark

Year Study Began: 2007

Year Study Published: 2017

Study Location: Two clinical centers in Denmark

Who Was Studied: Inclusion criteria were symptomatic varicose veins (Clinical–Etiological–Anatomical–Pathophysiological [CEAP] classification 2–6) with great saphenous vein (GSV) incompetence.

Who Was Excluded: Exclusion criteria were:
- Duplication of the saphenous trunk or an incompetent anterior accessory saphenous vein
- Small saphenous or deep venous incompetence
- Previous deep vein thrombosis
- Arterial insufficiency
- Tortuous GSV rendering the vein unsuitable for endovenous treatment

Patients: 500

Study Overview

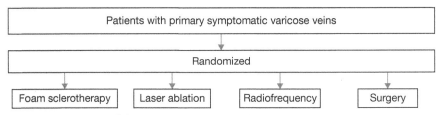

Figure 45.1 Design of the randomized controlled trial

Study Intervention: In this randomized controlled trial, patients were randomly assigned to undergo intervention for symptomatic varicose veins with ultrasound-guided foam sclerotherapy (UGFS), endovenous laser ablation (EVLA), radiofrequency ablation (RFA), or open surgery (HL/S).

Follow-up: 5-year analysis

Endpoints: *Primary outcome measures:* Ablated or absent GSV. An open refluxing segment of the treated part of the GSV of ≥10 cm at follow-up was considered a failure to strip or ablate the vein (technical failure). *Secondary outcome measures:* Presence of varicose veins during follow-up and the frequency of reoperations.

RESULTS

- A total of 500 patients (580 legs) were randomized to the four groups, with 125 (148 legs) in the RFA group, 125 (144 legs) in the EVLA group, 125 (145 legs) in the UGFS group, and 125 (143 legs) in the HL/S group. At 5-year follow-up there were 61 patients (68 legs) for analysis in the RFA group, 48 patients (53 legs) in the EVLA group, 42 patients (44 legs) in the UGFS group, and 55 (58 legs) in the HL/S group.

- Over 5 years, more patients in the UGFS group (31.5%) experienced a recanalization or experienced a failed stripping procedure versus 5.8% in the RFA group, 6.8% in the EVLA group (Kaplan-Meier estimate 6.8%), and 6.3% in the HL/S group.
- Fewer patients in the RFA group (18.7%) developed recurrent varicose veins than in the UGFS group (31.7%), EVLA group (38.6%), and HL/S group (34.6%).
- Within 5 years after treatment, 19 patients in the RFA group were retreated compared to 19 in the EVLA group, 25 in the HL/S group, and 43 in the UGFS group.

Criticisms and Limitations: A limitation of this study is the fact that it was not blinded, which may have resulted in bias impacting the perceived outcomes. While blinding patients to their assigned treatment may not have been feasible, it would have been possible to blind the observers in the follow-up period.

The study was not designed to investigate the long-term consequences of recanalization with regards to quality of life and clinical recurrence.

A relatively high number of patients did not show up for all follow-up visits despite a scheduled visit and a reminder letter. The 5-year analysis is based on less than half of the total population, which limits the long-term study results significantly and raises questions as to their validity.

In addition, the methodology of foam sclerotherapy used has been criticized by expert phlebologists as the technique and dosages were not optimal.

Other Relevant Studies and Information

- For patients with symptomatic varicose veins, the UK National Institute for Health and Care Excellence (NICE) guidelines recommend first offering endothermal ablation and endovenous laser treatment of the long saphenous vein, followed by UGFS and finally open surgery.[2]
- The European Society for Vascular Surgery recommends the use of endovenous thermal ablation techniques over foam sclerotherapy and open surgery.[3]
- The Society for Vascular Surgery states that endovenous thermal ablations (laser and radiofrequency ablations) are safe and effective, and recommends their use for treatment of saphenous incompetence. They recommend endovenous thermal ablation of the incompetent

saphenous vein over open surgery due to reduced convalescence and less pain and morbidity.[4]

• The Société Française de Phlébologie recommends that open surgery should only be offered on rare occasions.[5]

Summary and Implications: This trial demonstrates that for patients with symptomatic varicose veins with GSV incompetence, recanalization of the GSV occurred more frequently after UGFS, whereas no difference in the technical efficacy was observed in the other modalities in a 5-year period of follow-up. The higher frequency of clinical recurrence after EVLA requires confirmation in other studies. Based on this and other studies, major guidelines favor the use of endothermal ablation rather than UGFS, with surgery reserved for those with failed recurrent endovenous treatment.

CLINICAL CASE: MANAGEMENT OF PRIMARY GSV INCOMPETENCE

Case History
A 45-year-old female hairdresser is referred to your clinic with symptomatic primary varicose veins. She complains of heaviness, achiness, and itchiness. On examination, she has varicosities along the GSV distribution and the duplex ultrasound examination confirms an incompetent GSV, which is straight and subfascial in the thigh and suitable for endovenous therapy. How would the randomized controlled trial discussed in this chapter help you in offering a good option for this patient?

Suggested Answer
The trial discussed in this chapter showed that there was no difference in ablation rates between open surgery, EVLA, and RFA techniques. However, there were more clinical recurrences with EVLA compared to surgery and RFA. In view of the less invasive nature of the procedure, RFA might be the most suitable option for this patient.

References

1. Lawaetz M, Serup J, Lawaetz B, et al. Comparison of endovenous ablation techniques, foam sclerotherapy and surgical stripping for great saphenous varicose veins: Extended 5-year follow-up of an RCT. *Int Angiol.* 2017;36:281–288.

2. National Institute for Health and Care Excellence (NICE). Varicose veins: Diagnosis and management. 2013. https://www.nice.org.uk/Guidance/CG168

3. Wittens C, Davies AH, Bækgaard N, et al. Management of chronic venous disease: Clinical practice guidelines of the European Society for Vascular Surgery. *Eur J Vasc Endovasc Surg.* 2015;49(6):678–737.

4. Gloviczki P, Comerota AJ, Dalsing MC, et al.. The care of patients with varicose veins and associated chronic venous diseases: Clinical practice guidelines of the Society for Vascular Surgery and the American Venous Forum. *Vasc Surg.* 2011;53(5 Suppl):2S–48S.

5. Hamel-Desnos C, Miserey G. Varices saphènes et récidives: Traitements d'occlusion chimique ou thermique dans l'insuffisance des veines saphènes et des récidives. *Phlébologie.* 2018;71(3):10–17.

46

2-Year Results of a Multicenter Randomized Controlled Trial Comparing Mechanochemical Endovenous Ablation to Radiofrequency Ablation in the Treatment of Primary Great Saphenous Vein Incompetence

The MARADONA Trial

> The study suggests that [mechanochemical endovenous ablation] is a good alternative for treatment of great saphenous vein incompetence at 2 years of follow-up, although partial recanalization is more frequent than after [radiofrequency ablation].
>
> THE MARADONA INVESTIGATORS

Research Question: Is mechanochemical endovenous ablation (MOCA) as efficacious as radiofrequency ablation (RFA) in the treatment of primary great saphenous vein (GSV) incompetence?[1]

Funding: Vascular Insights Ltd.

Year Study Began: 2012

Year Study Published: 2019

Study Location: Four clinical centers in the Netherlands

Who Was Studied: Inclusion criteria were symptomatic varicose veins (Clinical–Etiological–Anatomical–Pathophysiological [CEAP] classification 2–5) with GSV incompetence.

Who Was Excluded: Exclusion criteria were:
• Active ulceration
• Previous surgery or treatment of the ipsilateral GSV
• Use of oral anticoagulants or known coagulation disorder
• Pregnancy or lactation
• Previous deep venous thrombosis or immobilization
• Contraindication or known allergy to sclerosant
• Severe renal or liver insufficiency
• Severe peripheral artery disease

Patients: 213

Study Overview

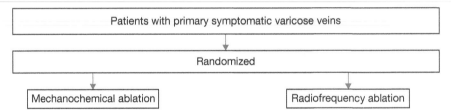

Figure 46.1 Design of MARADONA randomized controlled trial

Study Intervention: Patients were randomly assigned to MOCA without tumescent anesthesia or RFA.

Follow-up: 2-year analysis

Endpoints: *Primary outcome measures:* Postprocedural pain (evaluated using a 100-point visual analog scale during 2 weeks after treatment) and anatomic success at 1 year. *Secondary outcome measures:* Anatomic success, clinical success using the Venous Clinical Severity Score (VCSS), 30-day morbidity, disease-specific (Aberdeen Varicose Vein Questionnaire [AVVQ]) quality-of-life assessment, time to return to daily activities or work, reintervention rate, and any additional varicose vein treatment during 2 years of follow-up.

RESULTS

- The majority of patients were assigned to CEAP class C3 or C4a without baseline differences in VCSS and AVVQ scores between groups.
- Overall median pain scores during the first 14 days were significantly lower after MOCA ($p = 0.01$), although the absolute difference was small. At 30 days, similar numbers of complications and quality-of-life scores were observed. Hyperpigmentation was reported in seven patients in the MOCA group and two patients in the RFA group. The use of pain medication was similar, and there were no differences between groups in return to daily activities (Table 46.1).
- The 1- and 2-year anatomic success rates were lower after MOCA (83.5% and 80.0%) compared with RFA (94.2% and 88.3%), mainly driven by partial recanalizations, with the 1-year rate reaching statistical significance ($p = 0.025$).
- Median 30-day VCSS was significantly lower at 30 days after MOCA (1.0 vs. 2.0 in the RFA group; $p = 0.001$), whereas VCSS was comparable at baseline (MOCA, 4.0; RFA, 5.0; $p = 0.155$).
- Similar clinical success rates at 1 year (MOCA, 88.7%; RFA, 93.2%; $p = 0.315$) and 2 years (MOCA, 93.0%; RFA, 90.4%; $p = 0.699$) and no differences in health-related quality-of-life scores on the AVVQ at 1 year (MOCA, 7.5; RFA, 7.0; $p = 0.753$) and 2 years (MOCA, 5.0%; RFA, 4.8%; $p = 0.573$) were observed.

Table 46.1 2-YEAR OUTCOME STRATIFIED BY TREATMENT

	MOCA (n = 76)	RFA (n = 81)	p value
2-year anatomic success rate	80%	88.3%	0.066
2-year clinical success rate	93%	90.4%	0.699
Median time to fail, months	12.8	15.8	0.107
Improvement in VCSS	3 (2–5)	4 (3–5)	0.05
Reintervention at 2-year follow-up	3.9%	2.5%	0.675

Criticisms and Limitations

- The study stopped enrolling participants earlier than planned due to the suspension of reimbursement for MOCA treatment for CEAP C3 disease and lower. The study was therefore only able to recruit 46% of the calculated required number of participants and was significantly underpowered for the anatomic success outcome measure. The trial also consequently included a higher proportion of participants with more severe chronic venous insufficiency compared to other such trials.

• Although follow-up compliance was high, not all questionnaires were complete despite the best efforts of the trialists by offering evening and weekend follow-up visits.

• Bilateral treatment with MOCA is often not possible because of the maximum amount of sclerosant that can be used safely at one session, and therefore this might not truly represent real-world practice.

• Finally, as this is a new technique, there may be a learning curve for physicians practicing the MOCA procedure.

Other Relevant Studies and Information

• A randomized controlled trial by Vähäaho et al. compared MOCA with both RFA and endovenous laser ablation. The GSV occlusion rate 1 year after treatment was significantly higher after endovenous laser ablation and RFA than after MOCA. Quality of life was similar between interventions.[2]

• A recently published Cochrane Review concluded that there was a paucity of long-term data for MOCA.[3]

Summary and Implications: In this study, GSV ablation rates were lower after MOCA than RFA; however, both techniques were associated with similar clinical outcomes at 1 year and 2 years. MOCA resulted in more hyperpigmentation but less postoperative pain compared with RFA and a faster improvement in VCSS.

CLINICAL CASE: BILATERAL SYMPTOMATIC PRIMARY VARICOSE VEINS

Case History

A 38-year-old ward nurse is referred to your clinic with bilateral symptomatic primary varicose veins. She complains of heaviness and achiness and she does not like the aesthetic look of her legs. On examination, she has varicosities along the GSV distribution and the duplex ultrasound examination confirms bilateral incompetent GSV. The nurse has heard about the MOCA technique from colleagues in the veins clinic. How would you manage this patient?

Suggested Answer

This patient has symptomatic varicose veins bilaterally and should be offered intervention as part of the management for her varicose veins. The MARADONA study has shown both RFA and MOCA to have similar clinical outcomes at 2 years. However, the patient should be aware that there is a paucity of long-term outcomes after the MOCA procedure and there is a higher rate of pigmentation with it as well as lower GSV ablation rates. In addition, she would not be able to have both legs treated on the same day with MOCA. She opts for RFA treatment and makes an uneventful recovery.

References

1. Holewijn S, van Eekeren RRJP, Vahl A, et al. Two-year results of a multicenter randomized controlled trial comparing mechanochemical endovenous ablation to radiofrequency ablation in the treatment of primary great saphenous vein incompetence (MARADONA trial). *J Vasc Surg.* 2019;7(3):364–374.
2. Vähäaho S, Mahmoud O, Halmesmäki K, Albäck A, et al. Randomized clinical trial of mechanochemical and endovenous thermal ablation of great saphenous varicose veins. *Br J Surg.* 2019;106(5):548–554.
3. Whing J, Nandhra S, Nesbitt C, Stansby G. Interventions for great saphenous vein incompetence. *Cochrane Database Syst Rev.* 2021;8:CD005624.

SECTION 9

Vascular Access

JULIEN AL SHAKARCHI AND NICHOLAS INSTON

47

Multiple Preoperative and Intraoperative Factors Predict Early Fistula Thrombosis

The Hemodialysis Fistula Maturation (HFM) Study

[Early thrombosis] risk was higher in women than in men, for forearm than upper arm fistulas, for radial than brachial artery fistulas, and for fistulas constructed from smaller-caliber arteries or veins.

THE HFM INVESTIGATORS

Research Question: Do preoperative and intraoperative factors predict early thrombosis (ET) in newly created arteriovenous fistulas?[1]

Funding: National Institute of Diabetes and Digestive and Kidney Diseases

Year Study Began: 2014

Year Study Published: 2016

Study Location: Seven clinical centers in the US

Who Was Studied: Patients were included if they had current or anticipated need for maintenance hemodialysis within 3 months of arteriovenous fistula (AVF) construction and had placement of an autogenous single-stage AVF.

Who Was Excluded: Patients were excluded if they were aged >80 and not yet on maintenance dialysis, had a life expectancy of <9 months, or had anatomy unsuitable for autogenous AVF.

Patients: 602

Study Overview: This was a prospective observational cohort study of patients with newly created AVFs to identify preoperative and intraoperative risk factors for ET.

Study Intervention: Information was obtained preoperatively on demographic factors, comorbidities, and use of medications. Brachial artery flow-mediated dilation (FMD) and nitroglycerin-mediated dilation (NMD), arterial pulse wave velocity (PWV) measurement, and venous occlusion plethysmography were performed at baseline to assess vascular function. Duplex ultrasound was used to measure vessel diameters, flow rates, and arterial calcification. The surgeon's intraoperative assessment of AVF thrill (absent or extending to proximal, middle, or distal third of upper arm or forearm), expressed frustration (yes/no), and prediction of success (likely, marginal, unlikely) were also recorded. Postoperative serial duplex ultrasonography was performed within 3 days and at 2 and 6 weeks postoperatively.

Follow-up: Up to 4 years for overall study

Endpoints: Thrombosis was diagnosed clinically during postoperative visits and also at duplex ultrasound examinations. ET was defined as those cases that occurred within 18 days after fistula creation.

RESULTS

- The 602 participants had a mean age of 55.1 ± 13.4 years; 37% were >60 years old. 30% of participants were female, 44% were African American, 59% had diabetes, and 64% were on maintenance dialysis.
- ET was more common among women than men (7.7% vs. 4.7%) and in AVFs constructed from vessels 2.0–3.0 mm than from those >3.0 mm in diameter (arteries, 7.8% vs. 4.6%; veins, 8.5% vs. 4.5%) (Table 47.1).
- Age, BMI, smoking, hypercoagulability disorder, renal diagnosis, current maintenance hemodialysis, ipsilateral catheter use, and use of antithrombotic medications were not found to have a significant on ET.

- Only 2% of study participants with diabetes experienced ET compared with 10% of those without diabetes. Proportions of upper arm AVFs were similar for cohort members with and without diabetes.
- ET was associated with greater brachial artery NMD and with less trunk artery stiffness as assessed by PWV. The remaining measures of vascular function were not associated with ET.
- No associations of ET with subspecialty training of the attending surgeon or whether the attending or a trainee performed the anastomosis were found. The surgeon's intraoperative assessment of AVF thrill, expressed frustration, and prediction of success were all found to be significant predictive factors for ET.

Table 47.1 ET RISK DEPENDING ON RISK FACTORS

Risk factor	Number of patients	Odds ratio	95% confidence interval	p value
Female vs. male	327	2.75	1.19–6.38	**0.018**
BMI >30	230	1.19	0.53–2.70	0.67
Diabetes	360	0.19	0.07–0.47	**0.004**
Forearm vs. upper arm	225	2.76	1.05–7.23	**0.039**
Radial vs. brachial	225	2.64	1.03–6.77	**0.043**
Ipsilateral catheter use	155	0.99	0.11–8.55	0.99
No antithrombotic medications	230	1.23	0.52–2.93	0.63

Bold markings are significant results

Criticisms and Limitations: It is important to emphasize that the results from this study are only specific to ET and not failure to mature or to late thrombosis. The ET frequency was low despite a relatively large AVF sample size. Importantly, associations from such an observational study are vulnerable to confounders and hence can suggest but not imply causality.

Other Relevant Studies and Information

- The European Society for Vascular Surgery states in its vascular access guidelines that age and diabetes mellitus increase the risk of AVF failure. Interestingly, this was not found in the HFM study; to the contrary, diabetes was found to have a protective effect on ET.[2]
- The Dialysis Access Consortium study found a similar rate of ET (6%) compared to the HFM study (5.5%).[3]

Summary and Implications: ET was found to be associated with female gender and, unexpectedly, was relatively less common among persons with diabetes. Smaller-caliber vessels were also associated with poor outcomes. The surgeon's intraoperative assessment of thrill, expressed frustration, and fistula prognosis were each strongly associated with ET. The use of antithrombotic medication did not affect the rate of occurrence of ET.

CLINICAL CASE: AVF FOR DIALYSIS

Case History

A final-year medical student joins your theatre list. The next patient is a 65-year-old male listed for a left radiocephalic fistula creation. The medical student sees that the patient has been warned about the risk of ET. He asks how ET is defined and whether it can be prevented with an antiplatelet drug.

Suggested Answer

You explain to the medical student that ET is defined as loss of patency within the first 18 days after creation. It can be diagnosed clinically with loss of thrill and confirmed by an ultrasound scan. You ask him to read the HFM study reviewed in this chapter and he learns that the predictive factors found for ET in the study were female age, smaller arteries and veins, as well as the surgeon's assessment of thrill and fistula prognosis. He discovers that antithrombotic medications did not prove protective.

References

1. Farber A, Imrey PB, Huber TS, et al. Multiple preoperative and intraoperative factors predict early fistula thrombosis in the Hemodialysis Fistula Maturation study. *J Vasc Surg.* 2016;63(1):163–170.
2. Schmidli J, Widmer MK, Basile C, et al. Vascular access: 2018 clinical practice guidelines of the European Society for Vascular Surgery (ESVS). *Eur J Vasc Endovasc Surg.* 2018;55(6):757–818.
3. Lok CE, Moist L. More than reducing early fistula thrombosis is required: Lessons from the Dialysis Access Consortium clopidogrel fistula study. *Am J Kidney Dis.* 2008;52:834–838.

48

Long-Term Functional Patency and Cost-Effectiveness of Arteriovenous Fistula Creation Under Regional Anesthesia

A Randomized Controlled Trial

> These findings suggest that regional anesthesia has potential to improve [arteriovenous fistula] usage among the dialysis population, avoid complications of alternative access modalities, reduce surgical workload, and deliver cost savings to healthcare systems at large.
>
> AITKEN ET AL.

Research Question: Does regional anesthesia provide a benefit compared to local anesthesia on the long-term patency and cost-effectiveness of arteriovenous fistulas (AVFs)?[1]

Funding: None

Year Study Began: 2013

Year Study Published: 2020

Study Location: Three clinical centers in the UK

Who Was Studied: Patients >18 years of age undergoing creation of either a radiocephalic fistula or a brachiocephalic fistula for the purpose of hemodialysis were eligible for inclusion.

Who Was Excluded: Patients were excluded if they were unable or unwilling to provide informed consent, had undergone previous ipsilateral attempts at AVF creation, or had a radial or brachial artery of <1.8 mm or a cephalic vein of <2 mm at the wrist or <3 mm at the elbow during preoperative assessment. In addition, patients were excluded if they had an allergy to local anesthesia, significant peripheral neuropathy or neurologic disorder affecting the upper limb, infection at the anesthetic or surgical site, coagulopathy, or known ipsilateral central vein stenosis.

Patients: 126

Study Overview

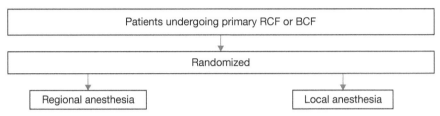

Figure 48.1 Design of randomized controlled trial

Study Intervention: Patients were randomly assigned to receive regional anesthesia (brachial plexus block; 0.5% L-bupivacaine and 1.5% lidocaine with epinephrine) or local anesthesia (0.5% L-bupivacaine and 1% lidocaine).

Follow-up: 12 months

Endpoints: *Primary outcomes:* Primary, functional, and secondary patency at 3 months. *Secondary outcomes:* Primary, functional, and secondary patency at 1 year.

RESULTS

- No patients were lost to follow-up. Six patients died during the follow-up period.
- Primary and secondary patency at 3 months were significantly higher in the regional anesthesia group than the local anesthesia group (84% vs. 62% for primary patency, p < 0.01) (Table 48.1).
- Primary, functional, and secondary patency at 1 year were also significantly higher in the regional anesthesia group than the local anesthesia group (79% vs. 59% for primary patency, p = 0.02).

- At 1 year, primary, functional, and secondary patency at 1 year were significantly higher in the regional anesthesia than the local anesthesia groups for radiocephalic fistulas (77% vs. 63% for primary patency, p = 0.02) but not for brachiocephalic fistulas (81% vs. 73% for primary patency, p = 0.36).
- Regional anesthesia resulted in estimated net savings of £195.10 (US$237.36) per patient at 1 year.
- In 12 months, 21 revisional procedures, 53 new AVFs, and 50 tunneled dialysis catheters were required.

Table 48.1 REINTERVENTIONS AT 1 YEAR

Procedure	Regional anesthesia	Local anesthesia
Superficialization/transposition	4	3
Collateral/branch ligation	2	0
Superficialization and collateral ligation	0	1
Revision of arterial inflow and collateral ligation	1	0
Distal revascularization and interval ligation	1	0
Proximalization	1	0
Radiologic declot and angioplasty	1	0
Outflow angioplasty/central venous stenting	6	1
New AVF	20	33
Arteriovenous graft	3	3
Tunneled dialysis catheter	21	29

Criticisms and Limitations: The study population is largely reflective of the UK population; hence, the results could be different internationally due to demographic differences.

The study is also limited by the lack of quality-of-life data as well as a lack of data on patient satisfaction of each procedure.

Cost-effectiveness is reflective of UK practice within the National Health Service and may not reflect practice in different healthcare settings.

Other Relevant Studies and Information

- Guidelines from the European Society for Vascular Surgery recommend that regional anesthesia should be considered in preference to local anesthesia for vascular access surgery because of a possible improvement in access patency rate.[2]

- The National Kidney Foundation's Kidney Disease Outcomes Quality Initiative (KDOQI) suggests that the choice of anesthesia for AVF creation should be based on the operator's discretion and best clinical judgment, as current evidence shows no difference between regional block or local anesthesia in terms of AVF usability, patency, interventions, or patient experience.[3]

Summary and Implications: The findings from this randomized controlled trial suggest that regional anesthesia, rather than local anesthesia, has the potential to improve AVF outcomes among the dialysis population, avoid complications of alternative access modalities, and deliver cost savings to the UK National Health Service.

CLINICAL CASE: ANESTHESIA FOR AVF CREATION

Case History

A patient is referred to your clinic for fistula creation. On ultrasound, the patient has a 2.5-mm cephalic vein at the wrist and a 2-mm radial artery on the non-dominant arm. You counsel the patient for the procedure and the patient asks which type of anesthesia will be used for the procedure.

Suggested Answer

You explain to the patient that the procedure is well tolerated under both regional and local anesthesia. There is evidence of published benefits for a fistula creation under regional anesthesia compared with local anesthesia with increased early (3 months) and late (1 year) patency rates and improves AVF usage.

References

1. Aitken E, Kearns R, Gaianu L, et al. Long-term functional patency and cost-effectiveness of arteriovenous fistula creation under regional anesthesia: A randomized controlled trial. *J Am Soc Nephrol.* 2020;31(8):1871–1882.
2. Schmidli J, Widmer MK, Basile C, et al. Vascular access: 2018 clinical practice guidelines of the European Society for Vascular Surgery (ESVS). *Eur J Vasc Endovasc Surg.* 2018;55(6):757–818.
3. Lok CE, Huber TS, Lee T, et al. KDOQI clinical practice guideline for vascular access: 2019 update. *Am J Kidney Dis.* 2020;75(4 Suppl 2):S1–S164.

SECTION 10

Trauma

JULIEN AL SHAKARCHI AND JACK FAIRHEAD

49

Durability of Endovascular Repair in Blunt Traumatic Thoracic Aortic Injury

Long-Term Outcome from Four Tertiary Referral Centers

In recent years there has been a paradigm shift from open repair to [thoracic endovascular aortic repair] as the preferred treatment for patients with blunt traumatic thoracic aortic injury.

STEUER ET AL.

Research Question: What are the early and long-term survival and reintervention rates in patients undergoing thoracic endovascular aortic repair (TEVAR) for blunt traumatic thoracic aortic injury?[1]

Funding: None

Year Study Began: 2001

Year Study Published: 2015

Study Location: Four clinical centers in Europe (one in Switzerland, three in Sweden)

Who Was Studied: All patients undergoing TEVAR for traumatic thoracic aortic injury at four tertiary centers between January 2001 and December 2010 were eligible for inclusion.

Who Was Excluded: Patients were excluded if they had died before the procedure could be attempted.

Patients: 74

Study Overview: This was a retrospective review of a prospectively held database of patients undergoing TEVAR for blunt traumatic thoracic aortic injury.

Study Intervention: All patients were initially managed according to the Advanced Trauma Life Support (ATLS) protocol. The initial evaluation was followed by computed tomography (CT) according to a trauma protocol. The aortic injury was characterized with respect to location, diameter, and length of the lesion, along with any concomitant injuries. In patients with concurrent injuries that were considered to be more life-threatening than that of the aorta, those were managed prior to TEVAR. Arterial access was established through open exposure or percutaneously. The stent-grafts were deployed over a stiff wire as per instructions for use. Oversizing of 15–60% was applied depending on device availability at the time of the trauma.

Follow-up: Minimum follow-up 2 years

Endpoints: The main outcome measures for the study were early and long-term survival, as well as complications and reinterventions.

RESULTS

- Nearly half of the patients (36 cases [49%]) had sustained the aortic trauma in association with a car accident. The second most common cause was a motorcycle or other motor vehicle accident, accounting for 16 cases (22%).
- The majority of the patients (64 cases [86%]) were treated within the first 24 hours of the trauma. Seven patients underwent TEVAR within the first week and the other three patients had delayed repair. In the whole cohort of 74 patients, one patient had a grade I injury, 10 (14%) had grade II injuries, 55 (74%) had grade III injuries, and eight (11%) had grade IV injuries.
- In all but two patients, one stent-graft was sufficient to seal the injured part of the aorta. The left subclavian artery was covered in 37 patients (50%), with only three patients subsequently requiring a left carotid–subclavian bypass. Four (5%) patients required coverage of the left common carotid artery (LCCA), which was managed by placing an LCCA chimney graft in

two patients and by a right-to-left carotid–carotid bypass in the other two patients.
- Early (30 day) mortality was 7/74 (9%), while 5-year survival was 81%. During follow-up after TEVAR, 13 (18%) patients underwent reintervention, half of them within the first month. The indications for reintervention were endoleak (n = 5), infolding (n = 5), left arm ischemia (n = 2), and fibrous hyperplasia (n = 1).

Criticisms and Limitations

- The study cohort was relatively small even though data were included from four tertiary centers over a 10-year period; therefore, it is difficult to draw robust conclusions. In addition, there are no results for patients who were managed medically or with open surgery.
- Another potential study limitation is that the stents used were different during the study period. Only a small proportion of those would have been newly developed devices currently available in the market.
- There are concerns over the long-term effect of cumulative radiation. There are currently no clear guidelines on follow-up protocols for this usually young cohort of patients.

Other Relevant Studies and Information

- Clinical practice guidelines of the Society for Vascular Surgery for endovascular repair of traumatic thoracic aortic injury recommend that endovascular repair should be performed over open surgical repair or nonoperative management. This should be carried out on an urgent basis within 24 hours of the injury if possible. It also suggests that magnetic resonance angiography may be preferable over conventional contrast CT angiography for long-term imaging.[2]
- The European Society for Vascular Surgery recommends that in patients with traumatic thoracic aortic injury with suitable anatomy, endovascular repair should be performed as the first option.[3]
- A 2020 published literature review concluded that TEVAR is considered the treatment of choice in blunt traumatic aortic injuries. In case of aortic rupture (grade IV) the treatment is mandatory, while intimal tear (grade I) and intramural hematoma (grade II) can be safely managed with nonoperative management. Debate is still ongoing on grade III (pseudoaneurysms) and whether they should be managed medically or surgically.[4]

Summary and Implications: TEVAR is a rapid, safe, and effective therapy in patients with blunt traumatic thoracic aortic injury. The initial outcome is highly dependent on the severity of other injuries, and most deaths are unrelated to the aortic injury once the stent-graft is in place. Patients with grade III and IV injuries should be considered for TEVAR.

CLINICAL CASE: SEVERELY INJURED TRAUMA PATIENT WITH THORACIC AORTIC INJURY

Case History
A 32-year-old female patient is admitted following a road traffic accident. Her Injury Severity Score is 30. The trauma CT scan shows a blunt thoracic aortic injury (grade IV) with no other life-threatening injuries. How would you manage this patient?

Suggested Answer
The patient requires an urgent TEVAR to stabilize the aortic injury. She should be transferred to the hybrid theatre with anesthetic cover for the procedure as soon as possible. A suitable stent with 20–30% oversizing should be selected. Following percutaneous access, the TEVAR is deployed over a stiff wire and coverage of the left subclavian artery is required to create a suitable proximal seal. The patient makes an uneventful recovery and does not require any reintervention in the first year following the procedure.

References

1. Steuer J, Björck M, Sonesson B, et al. Durability of endovascular repair in blunt traumatic thoracic aortic injury: Long-term outcome from four tertiary referral centers. *Eur J Vasc Endovasc Surg.* 2015;50(4):460–465.
2. Lee WA, Matsumura JS, Mitchell RS, et al. Endovascular repair of traumatic thoracic aortic injury: Clinical practice guidelines of the Society for Vascular Surgery. *J Vasc Surg.* 2011;53:187–192.
3. Riambau V, Böckler D, Brunkwall J, et al. Management of descending thoracic aorta diseases: Clinical practice guidelines of the European Society for Vascular Surgery (ESVS). *Eur J Vasc Endovasc Surg.* 2017;53(1):4–52.
4. D'Alessio I, Domanin M, Bissacco D, et al. Thoracic endovascular aortic repair for traumatic aortic injuries: Insight from literature and practical recommendations. *J Cardiovasc Surg (Torino).* 2020;61(6):681–696.

A Multicenter Trial of Vena Cava Filters in Severely Injured Patients

Early placement of a vena cava filter after major trauma did not result in a lower incidence of symptomatic pulmonary embolism or death at 90 days.

Ho ET AL.

Research Question: Do early vena cava filters provide a benefit to severely injured patients with contraindication to anticoagulation?[1]

Funding: Medical Research Foundation of Royal Perth Hospital, the Western Australia Department of Health, and the Raine Medical Research Foundation

Year Study Began: 2015

Year Study Published: 2019

Study Location: Three clinical centers in Australia

Who Was Studied: Patients aged ≥18 years were eligible if they had an estimated Injury Severity Score (ISS) of >15 and a contraindication to prophylactic anticoagulation within 72 hours of admission for the injury.

Who Was Excluded: Patients were excluded if there was imminent death, confirmed pulmonary embolism on admission, on systemic anticoagulation therapy before the injury, pregnancy, or unavailability of an interventional radiologist to insert the filter within 72 hours of admission.

Patients: 240

Study Overview

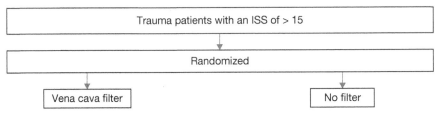

Figure 50.1 Design of randomized controlled trial

Study Intervention: Patients were randomly assigned to either a retrievable filter (vena cava filter group) within 72 hours of admission or no filter (control group). All filters were aimed to be removed as soon as prophylactic anticoagulation was established or before 90 days.

Follow-up: 30 days

Endpoints: *Primary outcome:* The primary endpoint was a composite of symptomatic pulmonary embolism (segmental pulmonary embolism on computed tomographic pulmonary angiography or by postmortem examination) or death from any cause at 90 days. *Secondary outcomes:* Symptomatic pulmonary embolism in the subgroup of patients who survived ≥7 days and who did not receive prophylactic anticoagulation within 7 days after injury, complications related to the vena cava filters, death at 90 days, major and nonmajor bleeding at 90 days, and deep vein thrombosis at 90 days.

RESULTS

- The median age was 39 years (interquartile range, 27–57). Of the 122 patients assigned to the vena cava filter group, 89% had the filter inserted within 24 hours after enrollment (median 15.6 hours [interquartile range, 3.0–22.3]).
- The composite primary outcome (pulmonary embolism or death at 90 days) was not significantly lower in the vena cava filter group compared to the control group (13.9% vs. 14.4%) (Table 50.1).

- Symptomatic embolism in the subgroup of patients who survived ≥7 days and did not receive anticoagulation occurred in five patients in the no-filter group compared to none in the filter group.
- The incidence of major and nonmajor bleeding, the incidence of deep vein thrombosis in a leg (11.4% of patients in the vena cava filter group vs. 10.1% in the control group), and transfusion requirements did not differ significantly between the two groups.
- The filter was not removed within 90 days in 37 patients, mostly due to technical reasons or loss to follow-up.

Table 50.1 PRIMARY AND SECONDARY ENDPOINTS

Outcome measure	Vena cava filter group (n = 122)	Control group (n=118)	Relative risk (95% confidence interval)
Composite of symptomatic pulmonary embolism or death from any cause at 90 days	17 (13.9%)	17 (14.4%)	0.99 (0.51–1.94)
Symptomatic pulmonary embolism among patients who did not receive anticoagulation within 7 days after injury	0/46 (0%)	5/34 (14.7%)	0 (0–0.55)
Death from any cause at 90 days	16 (13.1%)	11 (9.3%)	1.41 (0.69–2.87)
Major bleeding at 90 days	86 (70.5%)	78 (66.1%)	1.07 (0.9–1.27)
Nonmajor bleeding at 90 days	29 (23.8%)	21 (17.8%)	1.34 (0.81–2.2)

Criticisms and Limitations: The trial was designed on the basis that a sizable protective effect is needed to justify the initial costs, the risks of a vena cava filter insertion, and the additional cost of filter removal. Therefore, it might have been underpowered to detect small benefits.

The secondary outcome of systemic embolism introduced survivor bias as a patient had to survive to 7 days to qualify for inclusion.

Clinicians were not blinded and therefore decisions to start anticoagulation might have been affected by the presence of a vena cava filter. There was also a high number of exclusions (~70%), largely due to patients already receiving anticoagulants.

Other Relevant Studies and Information

- Guidelines offer conflicting recommendations on the use of vena cava filters for trauma patients.
- The Eastern Association for the Surgery of Trauma guidelines (2002) for the prevention of venous thromboembolism in trauma patients recommended that vena cava filters should be considered in high-risk trauma patients who cannot have anticoagulation.[2]
- The American College of Chest Physicians evidence-based clinical practice guidelines (2012) recommend that for major trauma patients, a vena cava filter should not be used for primary prevention of venous thromboembolism.[3]
- The Society of Interventional Radiology clinical practice guideline (2020) recommends against the routine placement of vena cava filters for primary venous thromboembolism prophylaxis in trauma patients without a known acute venous thromboembolism.[4]

Summary and Implications: Early prophylactic placement of a vena cava filter after major trauma did not result in a lower incidence of symptomatic pulmonary embolism or death at 90 days versus no placement of a filter. Therefore, use of a vena cava filter should not be considered routinely for trauma patients.

CLINICAL CASE: SEVERELY INJURED TRAUMA PATIENT

Case History
A 39-year-old male patient is admitted with multiple injuries following a road traffic accident. His ISS is 30. He is expected to be immobile for a period of time and due to his injuries cannot be anticoagulated for the next few days. The trauma surgeon asks if we should consider a vena cava filter for this patient.

Suggested Answer
This patient is at risk of a venous thromboembolism, but vena cava filters have not been proven to reduce the risk of pulmonary embolism or death at 90 days. Therefore, the patient would be exposed to the periprocedural risks as well as the risk of the filter not being removed within 90 days (34.5% of the filter group in the study) with no clear benefit. The patient should not have a vena cava filter and should be anticoagulated when it is safe to do so.

References

1. Ho KM, Rao S, Honeybul S, et al. A multicenter trial of vena cava filters in severely injured patients. *N Engl J Med.* 2019;381(4):328–337.
2. Rogers FB, Cipolle MD, Velmahos G, et al. Practice management guidelines for the prevention of venous thromboembolism in trauma patients: The EAST practice management guidelines work group. *J Trauma.* 2002;53:142–164.
3. Guyatt GH, Akl EA, Crowther M, et al. Executive summary: Antithrombotic Therapy and Prevention of Thrombosis, 9th ed: American College of Chest Physicians evidence-based clinical practice guidelines. *Chest.* 2012;141(Suppl):7S–47S.
4. Kaufman JA, Barnes GD, Chaer RA, et al. Society of Interventional Radiology clinical practice guideline for inferior vena cava filters in the treatment of patients with venous thromboembolic disease. *J Vasc Interv Radiol.* 2020;31(10):1529–1544.

INDEX

For the benefit of digital users, indexed terms that span two pages (e.g., 52–53) may, on occasion, appear on only one of those pages.

Tables, figures, and boxes are indicated by t, f, and b following the page number